The Coconut Oil Miracle
Health Benefits, Weight Loss, Recipes & More

Jenny De Luca

CONTENTS

ACKNOWLEDGMENTS

To the people who live in the areas where coconuts grow naturally who have known this for thousands of years and all the people who are trying to reintroduce this beneficial oil back into the West.

Introduction to Coconut Oil

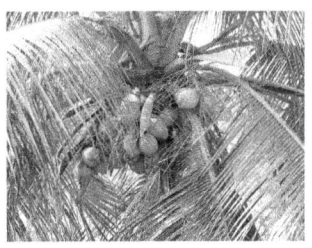 Coconut oil is an incredible oil that has been used by native people for thousands of years for health and beauty applications yet the West has remained largely ignorant of this amazing oil.

With the dramatic increase in preventable health problems and the insatiable quest for beauty, coconut oil has been recognized as having significant properties in both fields. It is amazing for your skin, can help clear up acne and it makes your hair look luxurious and silky. Not only that but it can help lower cholesterol, help you lose weight, reduce your blood pressure, aid digestion and reduce the signs of aging too!

It sounds almost too good to be true but Western societies are waking up to the natural health benefits that native people have been enjoying for thousands of years. Coconut oil has been embraced by the cosmetics and beauty industry and is now found in many lotions, potions, powders and creams as well as shampoo and conditioners.

Coconut oil is starting to find its way into foods and is slowly gaining popularity in cooking because that is one of the easiest and most convenient ways for you to gain the benefits of coconut oil.

Nowadays you can buy coconut oil easily online or you can find it in many health food shops and even larger supermarkets. With so many potential health benefits and beauty applications it is something you should buy right now and start using because it is going to help you so much!

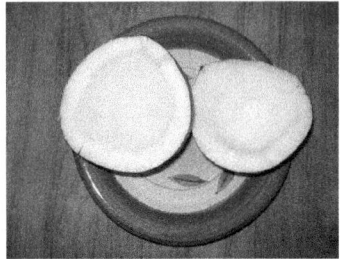

As you read this book you will learn all about coconut oil and how it can be used for everything from improving your skin to clearing up spots and helping your become a healthier person. Switching your cooking oil to coconut oil is going to have significant long term health benefits as well as reducing the effect of many complaints you could already be suffering from.

This book is a comprehensive guide to coconut oil and you will learn everything you need to know about it from where to buy it to which oil to buy to how to use it. You can start using coconut oil today and reaping the many benefits from it as it helps improve your health.

Whether you want to make your hair shiny, reduce the signs of aging, improve the quality of your skin or just boost your health, coconut oil can help you and you are going to learn all about this fascinating oil and how it is taking the West by storm with its many benefits and fantastic taste!

HEALTH BENEFITS OF COCONUT OIL

Coconut oil is one of those substances that is hailed by many people as a miracle oil because it is so beneficial to your health! As you read this book you will learn the many ways coconut oil can help you including:

- Skin care
- Hair care
- Stress relief
- Reducing cholesterol
- Boosting your immune system
- Aiding digestion
- Lowering blood pressure
- Weight loss
- Strengthening bones and teeth

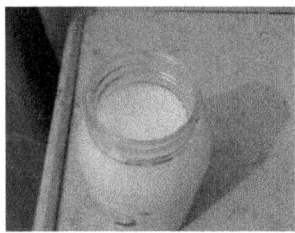

And of course much, much more. Many of the cultures who have a diet high on coconuts have low incidences of heart disease, cancer and other serious conditions which is down to the capric acid, caprylic acid and lauric acid which have antifungal, antioxidant, antibacterial and antimicrobial properties!

Coconut oil is very popular in tropical countries such as Thailand, India and the Philippines all of which produce their own coconut oil. In the West though it is not so popular, particularly after a successful war of propaganda by the corn/soy oil industries in the 1970s which sadly destroyed the popularity of this healthy oil.

Your body will take lauric acid and convert it into monolaurin which is helpful fighting both bacteria and viruses which cause diseases such as influenza, herpes and even HIV. It has also been shown to fight many types of harmful bacteria including listeria monocytogenes and the protozoa giardia lamblia.

Despite the many proven benefits, research into coconut oil is still in its infancy though it is popular in traditional medicinal systems such as Ayurveda, an India system of medicine.

Composition of Coconut Oil

Coconut oil is around 90% saturated fats, which is not as bad as you may think, and has traces of unsaturated fatty acids, monounsaturated fatty acids and polyunsaturated fatty acids.

The majority of the saturated fatty acids found in coconut oil are medium chain triglycerides which are easy for your body to assimilate. Around 40% of the total content is lauric acid with the rest being capric acid, caprylic acid, myristic acid and palmitic. The polyunsaturated fatty acids are typically linoleic acid and the monounsaturated fatty acids are oleic acid. Coconut oil also contains phenolic or gallic acid which gives the oil its aroma and taste. Virgin coconut oil is particularly strong in these polyphenols and so has a much more "coconutty" smell.

Hair Care

We'll discuss this in full detail later in the book but it is one of the best natural nutrients you can get for your hair, helping it to be shiny and grow well. It is very popular in India as a hair care supplement and leads to the luxurious thick and shiny hair often seen on people from this area who will apply the oil on a daily basis. Of course, it has many more benefits to your hair including dandruff prevention, head lice prevention and more.

Heart Disease

You would be forgiven for thinking that coconut oil is not good for your heart because it is high in saturated fats. However, because it is so high in lauric acid it is actually extremely good for your heart as it combats high blood pressure and high cholesterol levels. The saturated fats found in coconut oil are much better for you than those found in vegetable oils as they do not increase your LDL levels and helps look after your arteries.

Skin Care

Coconut oil is also a superb moisturizer and you will find out more about how it can benefit your skin, no matter what skin type you are. Think of coconut oil as being very similar to a mineral oil but does not have any adverse side effects and is perfectly safe. It helps reduce wrinkles and sagging, fighting the signs of aging as well as treating skin conditions such as psoriasis, dermatitis, eczema and others. If you look closely at the ingredients list of many of your skin creams you will find coconut oil in there somewhere!

Weight Loss

The short and medium chain fatty acids found in coconut oil are excellent for helping you get right of excess weight, being easy to digest and helping with the healthy function of your endocrine system and thyroid. It removes stress on your pancreas and boosts your metabolic rate, meaning you burn more calories.

Immune System

With the healthy acids found in coconut oil it works to support your immune system. Fighting viruses and bacteria it is excellent to keep your healthy and keep many of common diseases at bay.

Digestion

Using coconut oil also helps to improve your digestive system, particularly when used as a cooking oil as it can help prevent various stomach related issues such as Irritable Bowel Syndrome. The antimicrobial properties of the coconut oil helps combat parasites, bacteria and fungi that live in your digestive tract and stop them affecting you. It also helps your body absorb vital vitamins and minerals.

Candida

You'd be surprised how many people in the world suffer from candida, often without realizing, but coconut oil has been shown to prevent and even cure it. The oil provides relief both internally and externally and is a pleasant, gradual treatment meaning it is easy on your body. If using coconut oil to combat candida you should start with a smaller dose and build up rather than going straight for a larger dose.

Candida is surprisingly common across America and Europe due to the amount of yeast or fermented foods consumed and the general reliance on antibiotics which kill healthy gut bacteria. In the milder cases you have a sense of bloating but in more serious cases you can have inflammation, itching and more.

The capric acid, a medium chain fatty acid, reacts with other substances in your body to become monocaprin which is a powerful antimicrobial agent which will kill the yeast that causes Candida. All of the fatty acids in coconut oil have their role to play in fighting this complaint and it is surprisingly effective plus it doesn't have the side effects that many conventional medicines have.

Infections and Healing

Coconut oil is used for a wide variety of healing applications too, being very effective because it forms a layer that protects the infected area from air, dust, bacteria, viruses and bacteria. Coconut oil is great for bruises as it speeds up the healing process.

As coconut oil as antibacterial, antiviral and antifungal properties it is very effective in fighting numerous infections including hepatitis, herpes, measles, SARS as well as killing the bacteria that causes ulcers, urinary tract infections, gonorrhoea and pneumonia.

In research coconut oil has also proved effective in eliminating fungal and yeast infections such as thrush, diaper rash, athlete's foot and ringworm.

Other Health Benefits

We have just scratched the surface of the many health benefits of coconut oil and in itself these could make its own book, but at the end of the day it is incredible beneficial to your body. As well as all the above it has also been shown to assist with:

- Liver – the fatty acids help prevent liver diseases, prevent fat from accumulating in it and reduces the work load of your liver
- Kidneys – helps to dissolve kidney stones and prevent both kidney and gall bladder diseases
- Pancreatitis – coconut oil has been shown to be helpful in treating this condition
- Stress relief – applying coconut oil to your head together with a gentle massage will relieve mental stress
- Diabetes – coconut oil improves your body's production of insulin by helping to control blood sugar levels. It also helps your body effectively utilize blood glucose
- Bones – as coconut oil helps your body to absorb minerals, including

magnesium and calcium, it will help strengthen your bones. For women who are prone to osteoporosis coconut oil can be extremely helpful

- Teeth – Coconut oil helps your body absorb calcium which is going to help your teeth stay strong plus it has been shown to help prevent tooth decay
- HIV / Cancer – according to early research, coconut oil plays an important role in reducing the susceptibility to viruses for cancer and HIV patients plus it helps reduce the viral load of HIV patients
- Weight Loss – coconut oil is lower in calories than other oils and the fats are much easier for your body to convert into energy. Therefore the fats do not accumulate in your arteries or heart. Coconut oil is popular with athletes as it helps boost their energy and endurance, thereby enhancing their performance
- Alzheimer's Disease – according to new research coconut oil appears to be helpful in treating Alzheimer's and scientists are working to understand more about this

Common Coconut Oil Questions
When people first encounter coconut oil they usually have a few questions and these are going to be answered right now.

Why is coconut oil solid?
Coconut oil has a much higher melting point than most other oils commonly used in the home. It is solid at room temperature as it has a melting point of 76-78F or 24-25C. Most people when they buy coconut oil are surprised to find it is solid and think there is something wrong with it. Coconut oil does not need to be refrigerated.

How to use coconut oil?
For skin or hair care you just melt the coconut oil you want to use either by putting the bottle in the sun or in some warm water. Don't heat it in a microwave but you can melt it in a bowl over hot water if necessary.

Can I cook with coconut oil?
Yes, of course you can and it is very good for you! Just substitute coconut oil for whatever oil the recipe calls for. You can also mix coconut oil with other oils so you get the benefit of both, e.g. coconut oil and olive oil.

I don't like how coconut oil tastes
Try using the oil in different dishes that can disguise the taste of it until you get used to it. If it really makes you feel unwell then stop eating it as you

could well be allergic to it.

Coconut Oil Extraction Process

One of the most commonly used methods for extracting coconut oil is cold pressing and the other method is boiling fresh coconut milk. How the coconut is processed impacts the quality of the oil and because boiling will destroy many of the valuable nutrients this type of oil is considered a poorer quality than cold pressed oil.

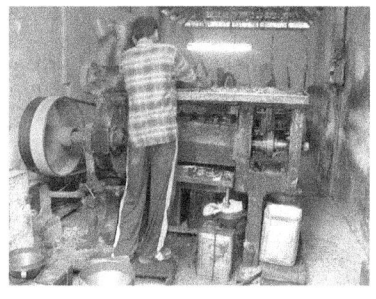

Cold pressing retains a much higher quantity of the goodness of the coconut and so you will get more health benefits from cold pressed oil. Typically coconuts are either machine or hand pressed. Most coconut oil is machine pressed purely because it is quicker and more economically viable. However, manual or bullock pressed coconut oil tastes better, has a better aroma and is unfortunately more expensive. Despite there being less manual pressed coconut oil on the market it is considered to be of a much higher quality.

Below you can see a picture of another coconut oil extraction plant.

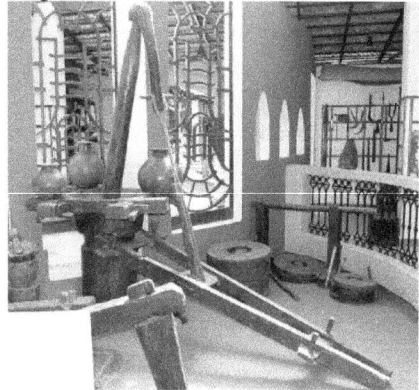

TYPES OF COCONUT OIL

There are five main types of coconut oil, each produced in a slightly different way and each having different properties. In this section you are going to learn the differences between the different types of coconut oil and how they can benefit you.

Virgin Coconut Oil
Virgin coconut oil is renowned for having a fantastic aroma, a great taste and being packed full of vitamins, antioxidants, medium chain fatty acids and many other beneficial things.

Virgin coconut oil is not just a fancy name given to coconut oil in order to "trick" consumers into buying it. It has some very important differences from normal coconut oil which are found in the source and extraction method. Because virgin coconut oil has more health benefits it is gaining popularity but can still be more difficult to get hold of.

Ordinary coconut oil is extracted by cold compression of the copra (dried coconut kernel) and has a moisture content of around 6%. Virgin coconut oil is extract from fresh coconut milk using processes such as fermentation, centrifugal separation and refrigeration to separate the soil from the water. Occasionally the resulting oil will be boiled to separate the oil and water further, though this will reduce the health benefits of the oil.

The reputable producers of virgin coconut oil will not heat the oil at any time during the manufacturing process, going to far as to keep the oil out of direct sunlight!

Virgin coconut oil has a slightly different appearance to normal coconut oil due to the presence of various colloidal and particulates. This oil should be almost as clear as water though there can be some color variation due to the production processes.

Virgin coconut oil is going to have a very strong fresh coconut smell and taste because it does come from fresh coconuts. As it is not refined all of the natural goodness of the oil is retained, including high vitamin E levels and minerals which are removed during filtration, refining and heating of normal coconut oil. The antioxidant and moisturizing properties of virgin coconut oil are much better than those of normal coconut oil.

Virgin coconut oil is higher in medium chain fatty acids, has good cholesterol and has virtually no trans fatty acids, making it much better for your body than regular coconut oil. If you are serious about gaining health benefits from coconut oil then this is the oil you have to use.

Normal coconut oil has almost no antioxidants in it because of the processing that takes place plus many of the vitamins and minerals are lost. Virgin coconut oil has a much longer shelf life than any other edible oil and does not go rancid very easily. It is very high in lauric and capric acid meaning there are significant health benefits from this oil and researchers are investigating the use of virgin coconut oil in treatment of a variety of diseases including AIDS.

Unfortunately, virgin coconut oil is more expensive than regular coconut oil because of the produced processes. The price will vary depending on the quality of the oil, the manufacturer and how much you are buying.

To buy this oil you will need to find a specialist health food shop or a larger grocery store. If they do not have it then there is a good chance they can order it in for you. Alternatively you can order it online but you need to make sure that you are getting what you pay for. You can of course find it on Amazon here though there are other places to obtain it from. Just ensure that you are buying pure virgin coconut oil as a few producers will add artificial flavoring to theirs.

The best virgin coconut oil comes from cold compression rather than fermentation. The latter has a much higher water content and will go rancid faster. If you are using the latter and need to melt it then do not put it directly on the heat but melt it in a cup of warm water.

Extra Virgin Coconut Oil

You will also hear about this type of oil and often see a premium being charged for it. However, according to the Asian and Pacific Coconut Community which sets the standards for coconut oils there is no such thing as extra virgin coconut oil. Typically the word extra is added on to the label to justify some extra cost to you!

Virgin coconut oil is considered to be the best of the coconut oils and if you really want to reap the benefits of using coconut oil then this is the one to use, though it is typically more expensive than the other oils but well worth it.

Unrefined Coconut Oil

Unrefined coconut oil is also known as crude coconut oil and is oil obtained directly from the coconut. It is unrefined, unfiltered and has no additives in it. You will hear it being called pure coconut oil which is used to differentiate it from bleached or refined oil. Virgin and organic coconut oils can be unrefined.

Unrefined coconut oil has a much better taste than refined coconut oil, retaining much of its original, natural taste. It will have a strong flavour of fresh coconuts which is lost in the refining process.

This coconut oil contains more nutrients than the refined variety and is richer in vitamins, antioxidants and proteins, which are virtually nil in refined oil. There is no chemical processing in this oil, whilst refined coconut oil is bleached and treated with sodium hydroxide. For anyone who is concerned about putting chemicals in their body this is ideal because it is much more natural.

However, because it does not undergo any refining, unrefined coconut oil can contain unwanted substances that are normally removed in the refining process such as dust particles. Its therapeutic uses are more limited than refined coconut oil plus it can be harder to get hold of. Because this oil is not refined it is considered less hygienic and therefore less suitable for any internal use.

Even though there is less processing in the production of unrefined coconut oil it is more expensive to buy purely because the majority of coconut oil is refined.

If you are using unrefined coconut oil for cooking then you need to ensure the oil is heated well to eliminate contamination. It should not be consumed raw and is best for external uses such as hair and skin. It is commonly used in the cosmetic industry.

Unrefined coconut oil is harder to buy but can be found in health food stores and larger grocery stores. Even though it is considered less hygienic it has still been used for centuries in the countries where coconuts grow naturally. The unrefined oil has a very positive effect on your skin and hair so is well worth using externally, perhaps with the virgin coconut oil for cooking.

Refined Coconut Oil

Whilst not necessarily the best or the purest coconut oil, the refined version is the most widely used variety, being known as RBD Coconut Oil or refined, bleached and deodorized coconut oil.

The oil that comes directly from the copra is often considered not fit for consumption because it can contain dust particles, bits of insect, microbes, fungal spores and other things that are not considered good for your health. This is down to how the coconut kernels are dried into copra.

The kernels are typically cut open and then spread out in the sun, with the flesh facing the sun, to dry. They are left like this for weeks or even months until they are dried and not covered with any form of netting. This means anything, and literally anything, can fall on them plus they get visited by birds, insects, rodents and who knows what else. Typically no cleaning takes place before they are processed so the oil is typically refined and cleaned before consumption.

After the oil is extracted (usually by hand or machine compression) it is filtered a number of times to obtain a clean liquid using calcareous clays. During this process the oil is bleached and then it is heated to a high temperature which kills germs and fungal spores whilst also deodorizing the oil. Then sodium hydroxide is added and the oil is filtered again to remove mono fats before it is hydrogenated which gets rid of unsaturated fatty acids so the shelf life is improved.

Refined coconut oil does not have the coconut smell or taste that you would get from pure oil. The deodorization is done because a lot of people really don't want the smell or taste of coconut in their cooking. Refined coconut oil has a much greater use in cooking because the dish will not end up with a coconut taste.

Whilst this oil is more hygienic than the unrefined oil it is not particularly beneficial for your health. Due to the processing there are almost no proteins and very few minerals left in the oil. On the plus side though the shelf life is longer.

This is the easiest of the coconut oils to obtain and is sold in most supermarkets and heath food shops. In fact most of the coconut oil that you see for sale will be refined coconut oil. If you only going to use coconut oil occasionally then this is a good oil to use because it will not spoil in your cupboard.

Pure Coconut Oil

This oil is well known for having a good aroma and taste as well as being packed full of antioxidants, beneficial vitamins and medium chain fatty acids. Pure coconut oil is used in cooking and cosmetics and is free from additives, flavorings, colors and more. It may or may not be refined but it will not be deodorized or bleached because these treatments involve a chemical process.

Pure refined coconut oil will have very little taste as the refining process will remove that but pure unrefined coconut oil will have a taste of coconuts about it. It can be hard to tell the difference and cheaper varieties can often be diluted with vegetable oils or flavorings. It is best to buy reputable brands where you know what you are getting.

Pure coconut oil has been used in cooking for centuries by people who live in coconut growing areas. It is a very stable oil and does not break down easily meaning it gives food prepared with it a great taste and aroma.

The pure oil is also easily absorbed by the skin, making it an ideal massage oil plus it is also very, very good for your hair! Pure coconut oil is used in a great deal of commercial cosmetics because it is so beneficial to your body. It is even used in some ointments and lotions as well as being used as a lubricant in some industrial machinery.

There are numerous health benefits from pure coconut oil, not least of which is that it will lower your bad cholesterol levels whilst raising the good cholesterol levels. It is great for your heart, helps to fight infection plus will make your skin and hair positively shine!

As it does not break down very easily it does not go rancid quickly and so is popular in culinary uses. It is not expensive to buy and you will get plenty of health benefits from using it.

Fractionated Coconut Oil

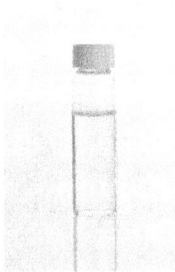

This type of coconut oil is the result of the search for a stable form of coconut oil that has a long shelf life and the beneficial qualities of coconut oil.

Fractionated coconut oil is the part of the coconut oil which has had the long chain triglycerides removed, leaving behind mostly medium chain triglycerides so it is a saturated oil, which gives it a long shelf life and increased stability.

The fractionating process will concentrate the levels of caprylic and capric acid which means the oil has a much strong disinfecting and antioxidant effect.

The oil is fractionated through a process of hydrolysis after which it is steam distilled to obtain the fractionated oil. Because this oil is both thin and stable it has a wide variety of uses, being used in cosmetics, as a carrier oil in aromatherapy, in medicines, for hair, for cooking and more.

Because there is a great deal more processing involved in the production of this oil it is going to be slightly more expensive but it does have a long shelf life, which means it is worth it. You can buy this from many health stores and supermarkets or you can get it online from companies such as Amazon here.

How & Where to Buy Coconut Oil

Before you buy coconut oil you need to decide what you are going to be used it for. Are you cooking with it? Using it for hair or skin? Using it in aromatherapy? For weight loss? With all the different varieties available you need to think carefully about which type of coconut oil you are going to buy.

To help you determine which variety is best for you here are some of the common applications of coconut oil and the best oils for them.

- Cooking – refined coconut oil
- Weight Loss – virgin coconut oil
- Carrier Oil – virgin coconut oil or fractionated coconut oil
- Heath Benefits – virgin coconut oil or organic coconut oil
- Massage – pure coconut oil or refined coconut oil
- Hair – pure coconut oil or refined coconut oil
- Medicinal Use – virgin coconut oil or organic virgin coconut oil

If you are using coconut oil for either therapeutic purposes or for cooking then refined coconut oil is better because it is more hygienic. Unrefined coconut oil is perfectly good for external use such as hair or skin care.

Most of the coconut oils can be found in larger health stores and supermarkets though virgin and organic coconut oil are much harder to get hold of but they can usually be specially ordered. If not then you can order them online which is often easier than visiting a number of different stores in attempt to find what you want.

There are numerous brands of coconut oil out there of varying quality but you should also read the ingredients carefully in case there are any additives and check the manufacturing date. Whilst coconut oil does have a long shelf life, fresh oil is still much better for you.

If you are buying online then it is worth reading the reviews on a site such as Amazon which will tell you which brands have a consistent high quality and which are of a lower quality. The more review, then the more information you have on that brand and whether or not they are worth buying.

The cost of coconut oil will depend on the type of coconut oil, where it comes from, how much refining took place and whether you are buying it online or not. Factors such as weather conditions and growing season in the coconut producing areas will also influence the price.

Although coconut oil has a long shelf life you do not want to buy huge quantities of it and have to store it. Fresh coconut oil is much better for you so typically you will only buy as much as you will use in a three to perhaps six month period.

Once you have opened your coconut oil you need to keep the lid firmly on the jar but it does not need to be refrigerated. Keep it out of direct sunlight and sources of heat and a typical sized jar will last for months.

So long as you determine what you are going to use your coconut oil for you will be able to buy the right oil for your needs. It is often best to buy it online purely from a convenience point of view.

Amazing Uses for Coconut Oil

Before we go into more detail about coconut oil let me introduce you to some of the interesting uses for it so you can start to really excited about this miracle oil and how you can use it in your life.

- Cuticle Care – rub coconut oil into your nail beds to treat dry or flaky cuticles and keep them in tip top condition
- Hair Care – there's an entire chapter dedicated to this but apply coconut oil directly to your hair, leave it for 40 minutes then rinse for shiny, well nourished hair plus rub the oil into the ends of your hair to stop them drying out
- Frizz Fighter – a little bit of coconut oil rubbed into trouble spots will repel moisture and help tame your hair
- Skin Conditioner – another subject with an entire chapter dedicated to it but mix coconut oil and baking soda and rub it on your skin in a circular motion to exfoliate and brighten your skin
- Face Mask – coconut oil and honey make for a very hydrating antibacterial face mask that in just 15 minutes will condition and tone your skin and help prevent spots
- Lips Nourishment – coconut oil and brown sugar make for a great lip scrub but just plain coconut oil is a great lip balm
- Exfoliant – coconut oil and salt or brown sugar makes for a very gentle but very effective exfoliating scrub for your skin
- Bath Oil – added to your bath water for a great moisturizing soak plus through in some Epsom salts to soothe your weary muscles
- Lip Tint – melt coconut oil with left over lipstick to produce a fantastic tinted lip balm

- Makeup Remover – a well-kept secret for removing heavy makeup; rub it into your skin, leave it for five minutes before wiping off with a warm cloth and it will remove any makeup! Use on a cotton wool pad to get rid of the most stubborn waterproof mascara
- Moisturizer – use coconut oil instead of your usual skin moisturizer and you'll find it sinks in really quickly plus leaves your skin really soft
- Shaving Cream – a fabulous shaving oil, particularly good for people with sensitive skin, as it helps you get a close shave and hydrates your skin
- Makeup Brush Cleaner – mixing coconut oil with antibacterial dish shop makes a superb brush cleaner
- Helps With Acne – coconut oil helps to reduce acne related inflammation as well as combating redness and irritating. Apply after cleansing your skin, best done just before bed
- Anti-Aging – helps to reduce the appearance of wrinkles and the signs of aging, being particularly good for the delicate skin around your eyes
- Dandruff Buster – massage coconut oil into your scalp to help fight dandruff
- Sunburn Oil – soothe painful sunburn with coconut oil to calm and moisturize your skin, helping to minimize peeling
- Eczema – helps to reduce itching and irritation
- Massage Oil – warmed coconut oil makes for a superb massage oil, particularly with a couple of drops of essential oil
- Deodorant – the antibacterial properties of coconut oil can help prevent the odor associated with sweating, though it is best used in addition to conventional products
- Tooth Polish – mixed with baking soda into a paste it is a great DIY toothpaste
- Foot Deodorizer – applied to your feet it helps to soften cracked and rough skin and deodorize at the same time (add some tea tree oil to the coconut oil first to help treat athlete's foot)
- Eyelash Strengthener – coconut oil on a cotton swab applied just before bed will help to strengthen those lashes
- Wax Remover – for the home waxer, coconut oil is a great way to get excess wax off your skin or any other surface you happen to get it on! Rub oil into the wax whilst it is still sticky and wipe it off with a warm cloth
- Shoe Shine – rubbing coconut oil onto patent leather is a fantastic way to bring back its high shine finish
- Chewing Gum Remover – coconut oil will remove tacky gum residue from any surface, including hair and carpet!

- Shower Cleaner – wiping your shower with coconut oil is a great way to keep it clean and wipe away shower scum
- Condition Wood – coconut oil is a great conditioner for wooden kitchen utensils plus it can be rubbed into wooden furniture to keep it looking fantastic
- Metal Cleaner – metal items that have lost their shine will benefit from being wiped with coconut oil. It's great for cleaning bronze and will also remove rush from steel!
- Hinge Oil – got a squeaky hinge? Lubricate it with coconut oil to stop the noise
- Guitar Care – coconut oil is great for conditioning and lubricating guitar swings
- Zipper Unsticker – a coat of coconut oil can help restore a stiff zipper back to full working order
- Leather Treatment – rub leather clothing or a sofa down with coconut oil to not only clean it but also to condition it and restore the shine
- Campfire Kindling – cotton wool balls soaked in coconut oil make a great kindling for a camper fire and is a lot safer than lighter fluid
- Motor Lubricant – use coconut oil as a lubricant on motors in your kitchen appliances or electrical items
- Cast Iron Seasoning – cast iron kitchen items need seasoning before you can use them and coconut oil is one of the best ways for you to do this
- Hairball Help – coat your cats paws with a little oil to stop him or her from coughing up hair balls
- Fur Conditioner – rubbing coconut oil into the coat of your dog or cat will help keep it healthy and shiny, just like it does your hair
- Food Supplement – a little coconut oil into your pet's diet can help improve their heath from weight control, doggie breath and even arthritis protection
- Soothing Balm – rub coconut oil into itchy spots to help relieve the irritation
- Tea and Coffee Additive – use to sweeten your drink instead of sugar or honey
- Nut Butter – make your own fresh nut butter and gain even more of the benefits of coconut oil
- Cooking – use instead of vegetable oil for a great taste to your dishes, plus it is brilliant for roasting vegetables or scrambling eggs; more on cooking with coconut oil later in the book
- Salad Dressing – adds to the flavor of your salad, giving it a more

unusual taste

- Granola – a fantastic ingredient to any granola that gives it a really interesting taste – more on this in the recipe section
- Toast Topper – use instead of butter on your toast with a sprinkle of cinnamon … delicious!
- Smoothie Ingredients – add to a smoothie for a coconut taste, extra energy and health benefits
- Baking Ingredient – fantastic in baking instead of butter, vegetable oil or shortening
- Popcorn Oil – coconut oil is brilliant for popping corn in as it gives the corn a sweet, slightly coconutty taste
- Pan Greaser – instead of greasing your pan with vegetable oil or lard use coconut oil
- Mouthwash – swill your mouth out with coconut oil for three to five minutes for whiter teeth and fresher breath
- Colds and Flu – coconut oil boosts your immune system and boosts your white blood cell count so is great to prevent you getting ill and fighting any illnesses you do get
- Chafing – not only does it prevent chafing but it also soothes any areas that are chafed! Great for babies who suffer from diaper rash too
- Sore Throat – swallowing a little coconut oil is great for a sore throat or brilliant when added to your tea
- Headlice – rinsing your hair in apple cider vinegar, drying it and then brushing through coconut oil, leaving for 24 hours before rinsing will help get rid of head lice
- Cold Sore Treatment – apply coconut oil the second you feel the tingle of a cold sore where its antiviral properties will help prevent the cold sore
- Scrapes and Scratches – apply a thin layer of coconut oil over a scratch or scrape (not a deep wound) to act as a barrier and keep out bacteria and dirt
- Bug Bites – a couple of drops gently rubbed in will relieve the itching
- Bruising – rub into bruises helps to reduce inflammation and heal the bruise
- Yeast Infections – applied topically and ingested some people have found that coconut oil helps to treat yeast infections
- Cholesterol – coconut oil boosts your good cholesterol whilst reducing your bad cholesterol
- Stomach Calmer – helps to soothe your stomach, particularly useful if you suffer from ulcers, Crohn's Disease or irritable bowel syndrome

- Congestion – mixed with tea tree and rosemary oil you rub this on your chest and under your nose to help clear your sinuses
- Insect Repellent – coconut oil combined with peppermint, rosemary or tea tree oil makes for an excellent insect repellent
- Dry Noses – coconut oil is great to help keep your nostrils moisturized which can prevent nosebleeds
- Breastfeeding Help – any new mother will tell you about painful or cracked nipples from breastfeeding and coconut oil helps keep them moisturized and stop this from happening
- Metabolic Booster – using coconut oil in your diet will help your liver function and encourage your body to burn fat

Coconut oil has a whole multitude of different uses and as you continue through this book so you will find out more about how this miracle oil can benefit you.

COCONUT OIL FOR BEAUTY

The cosmetics industry is a heavy user of coconut oil and you will find it in many beauty products where it is valued for its moisturizing properties and being high in antioxidants and other minerals. Many of the products you buy off the shelf will have coconut oil in and for many it is promoted as being beneficial, which it is, but you can skip the chemicals and just use the coconut oil to reap those benefits without the expense of creams and lotions!

Some of the best home uses for coconut oil include:

- Makeup Remover – rub it on directly or using a cotton pad to get rid of even the most waterproof makeup
- Body Lotion – coconut oil is great in pretty much any body lotion as it is so moisturizing
- Cuticle Oil – don't buy the expensive oils in the stores, just use some coconut oil instead at the base of your nails
- Lip Balm – brilliant for chapped lips and keeping your lips moisturized
- Stretch Mark Cream – rub into your belly to help prevent stretch marks from forming and also to prevent blisters and dark spots forming
- Under Eye Cream – dab coconut oil under your eyes to help combat bags and fine lines
- Body Scrub – half a cup of coconut oil and a handful of brown sugar or coarse salt (try Himalayan pink salt) makes for a superb exfoliator with moisturizing action!
- Dandruff Treatment – massaging coconut oil into your scale stimulates hair growth and combats dandruff … much better than chemicals
- Body Oil – coconut oil makes for the best moisturizing body oil and is naturally SPF 4!

- Night Cream – apply coconut oil to your face / neck just before bed and it will smooth fine lines and wrinkles as you sleep
- Foundation Primer – coconut oil is the perfect primer for your foundation, just let it soak in to your face and then add your foundation, which will look smooth and stay on longer

There are lots and lots of things you can do with coconut oil but let me share with you three of my favorite face mask recipes. These are superb for your skin and easy to make.

When making a face mask the best coconut oil to choose is unrefined, organic, cold pressed virgin olive oil as it does not contain any additional ingredients and is much less likely to cause any allergy problems. If you have any concerns about being allergic to coconut oil, try it on a small part of your skin to see how it affects you.

Honey and Lemon Face Mask

Coconut oil has a very small molecular structure and so it can get in to your skin and soften it from the inside. Honey is excellent at hydrating your skin and the lemon is a natural astringent which tightens your skin and shrinks large pores.

Honey is well known for its antibacterial and antiseptic properties and is used to combat acne and pimples. It's a great exfoliator and helps to face scars and blemishes.

Ingredients:
- 1 tablespoon coconut oil
- 2 tablespoons raw honey
- ½ teaspoon lemon juice

Method:
1. Mix the ingredients well in a small bowl
2. Apply generously to your face (clean your face first)
3. Leave for ten minutes before rinsing off with cool water
4. Pat your face dry with a soft towel

Banana and Turmeric Face Mask

This face mask is superb for fighting acne and moisturizing your skin. Coconut and turmeric are great for their anti-inflammatory properties whilst the banana is very hydrating, fighting wrinkles, reducing scarring and smoothing out rough skin. The turmeric is well known for its anti-aging properties and is also antiseptic and antibacterial, meaning it is ideal for your skin. It helps combat acne and brightens dull skin.

Ingredients:
- 1 tablespoon coconut oil
- ½ ripe banana (overripe is best)
- Pinch of turmeric (it won't stain your face but may stain your fingernails so use a nailbrush and lemon juice to get rid of it.

Method:
1. Mash up the banana in a small bowl
2. Stir in the coconut oil and turmeric until it is evenly distributed
3. Apply the face mask to your clean face and leave for 15 minutes
4. Rinse with cool water and then pat your face dry

Nutmeg and Avocado Face Mask

This is a wonderful face mask because the avocado protects your skin against free radicals, helping to slow down the signs of aging whilst moisturizing and hydrating your skin. The nutmeg is an exfoliant and will help to prevent breakouts.

Ingredients:
- 1 tablespoon coconut oil
- ¼ ripe avocado (mashed into a smooth paste)
- ½ teaspoon ground nutmeg

Method:
1. Mix the ingredients together in a small bowl until it is evenly mixed
2. Apply generously to your face using a circular motion
3. Leave for around 15 minutes
4. Rinse off with cool water then pat your face dry with a clean towel

Coconut Oil for Acne

Coconut oil is actually very effective in treating acne and is very beneficial for anyone who suffers from this uncomfortable condition. Acne is a common problem, mostly found in teenagers though it can affect adults of any age. Typically once puberty has passed the acne will clear up but it is still painful and awkward and can leave permanent scarring. For some people getting rid of acne is easy but for others it takes a lot more work and it is a subject of its own numerous books but coconut oil can be very useful for anyone of any age struggling with acne.

Acne is caused by an infection in the sebum glands which are on the skin and secrete oils to prevent your skin from drying up and cracking. These glands get clogged and bacteria grows which means that the sebum secretion is obstructed and so you get redness, inflammation, swelling and pain.

Acne is worse in teenagers because due to the hormonal changes in their body the sebum production is increased significantly, which results in oily skin and sometime pimples, spots or even minor acne. With the help of various soaps, lotions and other chemicals they can help keep it at bay but that doesn't stop the oily secretions and it removes the antimicrobial guard from the skin. This means the pores are effectively defenseless to infections and so bacteria invades, blocks the sebum glands and acne appears.

There are a number of components in coconut oil which help combat acne including:

- Fatty Acids – coconut oil contains lauric acid and capric acid which are two very powerful antimicrobial agents. These acids are found in breast milk and help to protect new born babies from infections. When applied to your skin these acids are converted into monocaprin and monolaurin which then provide a protective layer which helps prevent the bacterial infection. Direct application is best but even consuming coconut oil will provide some relief.

- Vitamin E – this vitamin is very important for healthy skin and proper functioning of sebum glands, clearing any blockages. It is treats the root cause of acne rather than just the symptoms. Vitamin E can also help balance the hormonal fluctuations that lead to overactive sebum glands.
- Anti-Inflammatory – coconut oil has very small molecules and so it penetrates easily and deeply into the skin, being absorbed very quickly. It will almost immediately start reducing inflammation from acne and help provide a protective barrier over any open wounds. It improve your metabolism which helps balance hormones and reduce acne, also repairing damaged skin cells.

You can make up a wide variety of different products with coconut oil such as the face masks discussed in the previous chapter or just apply coconut oil directly to your skin. Even eating up to five tablespoons of the oil a day, which isn't unpleasant, will help reduce your acne. For best results add coconut oil to your diet and apply it two or three times a day to your face.

You want a very high quality coconut oil to use on your skin. The unrefined variety is considered unhygienic and could contain dust which will clog your pores. The best choice is refined virgin coconut oil which, whilst more expensive, is absolutely ideal for your skin!

Coconut oil is classified as a light microbial agent meaning that against the more serious cases of acne it cannot be your only treatment. For medium or light cases you can use coconut oil and get excellent results. For the more serious cases you need to talk to your physician and combine coconut oil with other treatments.

Remember though that results will vary from person to person and that you need to look at all aspects of your life, including diet, hygiene, sleeping and more in order to truly clear your acne. Coconut oil is considered an excellent treatment for acne and will definitely provide relief and help with it.

COCONUT OIL FOR HAIR

Coconut oil is one of the best hair oils that you can get and is used not only by people in the countries where coconuts grow but across the world too. Many of the Western hair care products contain coconut oil because it is so good for your hair, making it shiny and strengthening it.

Coconut oil has been used as a hair oil literally for thousands of years and produces remarkable results. It is full of vitamins, minerals and carbohydrates which are very beneficial to your hair plus it has a strong moisturizing and conditioning effect. It has been shown to help prevent hair loss and baldness by encouraging strong and healthy hair growth.

In India coconut oil has been used since time immemorial for hair grooming and to prevent hair loss. Boiling leaves in coconut oil is excellent for preventing hair loss. Massage this into your scalp and it will help improve the quality of your hair too. Another traditional hair loss recipe is lime water and coconut oil or coconut oil and gooseberries (boil the gooseberries in the oil). Both of these have been used to prevent hair loss and appear to be effective.

With many people in the West drying their hair, coloring it and using straighteners it causes damage to your hair which is why a lot of people buy expensive products that restore protein to hair and help it look good. Coconut oil helps to reduce protein loss in your hair and the lauric acid easily penetrates the hair shaft. Coconut oil can be put on your hair before or after you wash it plus massaging it into the scalp helps to stimulate hair growth and prevent dandruff.

Another advantage of coconut oil is that it helps your hair to retain moisture, which helps to prevent frizz and breakage. Coconut oil is very stable and does not break down easily so it does not let valuable moisture escape from your hair.

Coconut oil is a far better conditioner than anything you can buy on the shelves in your local supermarket. An application of warm coconut oil will help keep your hair soft and shiny. Just brush it through your hair at night then wash it out the next morning, repeating every few days.

The uses of coconut oil in hair just go on because it also makes a good styling oil because it melts when warm and then solidifies as it cools. When you apply it to your hair it will thin and spread and then condense as it cools, making it ideal for styling your hair!

Head lice are a common problem in many children and tend to keep on coming back. There are chemical products available but these often have limited effect and can damage the hair or scalp. Coat the hair with coconut oil and then comb with a lice comb and you will find it so much easier to run the comb through the hair and get the lice out.

Dry hair is a problem many people suffer from and spend a lot of money on products to help combat the issue. However many of the products that are used to treat dry hair can end up causing scalp damage and dandruff. Coconut oil is highly moisturizing and very good for dry hair.

Apply a warm mixture of lavender oil and coconut oil to your hair and scalp before bed, then wash it out in the morning. This is a superb toner for your hair and will help improve the quality of your hair. You can do this every day or even every couple of days and your hair will become softer, shinier and more full bodied.

Coconut oil can be used as a conditioner which is obviously very effective. A paste made of henna, warm milk and coconut oil applied for the hair for twenty minutes before rinsing is a very effective conditioner, particularly for anyone who suffers from dry hair.

Another common problem is split ends and the usual solution is to cut the split ends out, which often means losing more hair than you want. Massaging your hair with a mixture of almond and coconut oil will help reduce the chances of split ends and help join them back together.

Coconut oil is a traditional remedy for baldness, grey hair and thinning hair. Mixed together with Eclipta Alba or Bhringraj leaf juice or even just used by itself it can help strengthen the hair and stimulate hair growth.

The cosmetics industry has worked out how important natural oils such as coconut oil is to your health and wellbeing as you will see these oils included in many store bought shampoos and conditioners. For some reason people in the West view applying oil to the hair as primitive yet the results are startling and cannot be ignored.

With so many chemicals used on hair as well as drying and other tools a lot of people have very damaged and weak hair. Regularly oiling your hair with coconut oil only takes a few minutes but it protects your hair from the ravages of beauty products and keeps it looking fantastic. If you doubt this then try using coconut oil in your hair for two weeks and see the difference; take before and after photos and you will see just how much of an improvement there is.

The fact that major corporates are using natural oils like coconut in their products and using this as a selling point tells you that this is very effective yet you can bypass the cost and the chemicals by just using coconut oil directly.

Coconut oil is incredibly good for your hair and you only have to look at the cultures that regularly use it in their hair to see just how good it is. Think of the Pacific Islanders or Asian cultures where coconut oil is regularly applied to their hair … they have thick, strong, luxurious hair and their secret is a natural product you can easily get hold of!

Coconut Oil for Skin

Coconut oil is widely used throughout the cosmetics industry and because of all the properties described earlier it is excellent for your skin and is even used as a sun cream in the areas where coconuts grow naturally.

Coconut oil is high in saturated fats which are mostly medium chain fatty acids also known as triglycerides. These help keep skin smooth and because coconut oil is high in these fats it helps your skin to retain moisture. As you use coconut oil in your cooking so these triglycerides are deposited under the skin, helping to give it an even town and reducing the appearance of wrinkles and pores.

You will also find high concentrations of lauric, caprylic and capric acid in coconut oil which have strong antimicrobial and disinfectant properties which means they protect the skin from microbes that can get into wounds or go through your pores. This works whether you consume coconut oil or just apply it externally.

These three acids are easily broken down into energy which means they can provide you with a significant boost to your energy levels before you work out which is why they have been linked to weight loss. When you lose weight you often improve the quality of your skin and working out means you tone the muscles beneath the skin.

Vitamin E is well known as being beneficial to skin, which is why many skin creams contain it. It is important for protecting your skin from cracking, skin growth, smooth skin and repairing the day to day wear and tear of your skin. Perhaps most importantly vitamin E is a good antioxidant and so fights free radicals which cause the signs of aging and wrinkling. In 100g of coconut oil you will find approximately 0.1mg of vitamin E. Coconut oil is well known for its ability to reduce the signs of aging and can be found in many expensive anti-aging creams.

Coconut oil is very rich in proteins which help to rejuvenate your skin and keep it healthy. These proteins help your body repair damaged tissue and keeps your cells healthy. Coconut oil can help reduce the signs of scarring and stretch marks because it feeds the skin.

Best of all, when you apply coconut oil to your skin it is not going to go rancid. Many other oils will go off after a while on your skin, often just a short while, leaving a peculiar smell. Not coconut oil though ... plus you have a tropical smell about you too!

Coconut oil makes for an excellent lip gel which is free from potentially harmful chemicals. Just rub some on your lips and they will shine, be moisturized and look fantastic!

If you use expensive lotions and creams to soften your skin then you will be pleased to know that coconut oil is fantastic for your skin. If you have hard or dry skin just put some coconut oil on your palms, rub them together a couple of times and then apply the coconut oil to wherever you want to moisturize.

If you suffer from cracked or dry feet or hands then coconut oil is ideal. Whilst it will not get rid of cracks in your feet it will definitely soften your feet and ease any discomfort.

Coconut oil is great when mixed with exfoliating substances like salt or sugar and can really enhance their effects. Not only will you remove the dead skin but you will leave your skin moisturized and feeling soft and smooth!

As we mentioned before coconut oil makes an ideal make up remover because it can get even the most stubborn make up off your face. However, what we didn't mention is that coconut oil is perfectly natural and moisturizing to your skin meaning that you are not going to damage your skin, get it in to your eyes and so on like you often do with make-up remover which can be painful!

Skin complaints such as psoriasis and eczema can be helped with coconut oil and research is underway to validate these claims. However, because coconut oil is very moisturizing and high in important proteins it can help replace and repair damaged or dying cells. With its antibacterial properties it can also fight any potential infection whilst also reducing any visible marks on the skin. If you suffer from any skin complaints then try coconut oil on a small area of your body and a week or two and see how different it is. Unfortunately the conventional medicine approach precludes the use of natural and healthy solutions such as coconut oil, eschewing them for expensive chemical laden products that line the pockets of the big pharmaceutical companies.

Coconut oil isn't difficult to use and for beauty applications externally you can use an unrefined oil. It is better to buy a jar that has a wide neck because it is easier for you to get your hands in. Coconut oil, as you know, comes as a solid so you will either have to warm it slightly or melt it in your hands by rubbing your palms together before applying it. You can rub cotton pads in your coconut oil and then rub them on your body which will also melt the oil. You do not need a lot of coconut oil to create a protective shield for your skin.

Remember that your skin can only absorb so much coconut oil so don't use too much. If your skin ends up looking oily, shiny or greasy then you may well have applied too much which can make a mess of your clothes!

Using a little coconut oil regularly on your skin will significantly improve its quality, moisturize it and help keep it looking fantastic. It will do all of this naturally and when you consider how much cheaper coconut oil is than even the cheapest anti-aging cream then you will realize just how effective and useful it is.

Coconut Oil Capsules

One of the obsessions of the West is to put anything healthy into a capsule. It makes it look sterile and clean, ensuring it is easy for you to take with the minimal of fuss and effort. Our whole culture is about convenience and speed, with the benefits of coconut oil trying to be squeezed into a capsule.

For anyone who is busy or wants the benefits of coconut oil without the hassle of a jar of solid oil on the shelf then capsules are ideal. Whilst they are portable and easy to take they do not have all of the benefits of coconut oil, but they do have most of them!

Typically the capsules are a concentrated coconut oil extract shoved into a starch capsule that is easy for you to take. Some of these capsules are supplemented with other vitamins, medicines or herbal substances whilst others will be pure, refined, virgin or organic coconut oil, though after all that refining the latter can be doubted.

You can often find organic and virgin coconut oil in soft gel tablets with a recommended dose of 4 to 6 capsules a day. Whilst these are great a lot of people struggle to swallow these soft capsules.

The advantage of capsules is that they are easy to take and easy to carry around with you. You can manage your doses very precisely because the quantities of vitamins in each tablet is a known quantity. In capsule form coconut oil is good for weight loss, treating candida, treating hair loss, reducing your bad cholesterol whilst increasing the good cholesterol, boosting your metabolism, treating digestive problems, maintaining healthy skin and fighting microbial infections.

Coconut oil capsules can often be cheaper than buying coconut oil as you can see from here. You can buy a month's supply of tablets (120) for under $9 which is a good price and certainly cheaper than coconut oil. If you are keen on gaining the benefits of coconut oil then using the capsules as well as using the oil in your cooking is a good way to really ensure you get the most from this miracle oil.

Coconut oil capsules have become popular because people demand pills; they are convenient, easy to take and require absolutely no effort. Manufacturers know there is a market for coconut oil in this form and so they produce the capsules and enjoy the profit!

However, these capsules do not contain all of the benefits of coconut oil because they are highly processed the taste and flavor are removed but they also lack the natural, pure component of the oil. Many of the volatile nutrients are lost in processing and heating which means you miss out on a great deal of the benefits.

Whilst you may think that capsules are a good idea they can end up working out far more expensive than regular coconut oil. Many experts recommend a daily dose of around 50g of coconut oil, bearing in mind a tablespoon is 15g. A single coconut oil capsule will typically contain around 1000mg of coconut oil, meaning you have to consume a vast amount of capsules to get the same dose!

Soft gel capsules are also often made from animal gelatine, meaning they are not suitable for vegans and many vegetarians. If you prefer organic produce then you need to ensure that the gelatine itself is organic.

In my opinion coconut oil capsules are better than nothing. If you haven't got the time to cook with coconut oil or can't face spooning some from the jar then capsules are a good fall back. They are also an excellent addition to your diet if you are cooking with coconut oil to ensure you get plenty of the oil. Whilst it doesn't have all the vitamins and minerals found in coconut oil it is better to take a capsule than not to take any coconut oil at all.

COCONUT WATER BENEFITS

We will just step away for a moment from coconut oil and look at coconut water which is found in the center of the coconuts you buy at the store. Like the oil, the water is full of benefits, being great for digestive problems, protects your heart, lowers bad cholesterol levels and more. Coconuts really are a miracle fruit with the flesh itself being packed full of nutrients and energy.

Coconut water contains protein, fat, carbohydrates, sugars, fiber and plenty of vitamins and minerals that are vital to a healthy functional body. It is a very energy dense food, making it ideal for athletes and people who work out a lot.

Coconut water can be drunk to rehydrate your body because not only is it water but it is full of minerals and vitamins including potassium and sodium which are important electrolytes. A glass or two of coconut oil after being out in the sun can help rehydrate you and re-energize you as you regain the minerals and vitamins you lost during the day.

Coconut water is also pretty good for almost any digestive disorder including diarrhoea, flatulence, vomiting, gastroenteritis and more. Coconut water, like the oil, has strong antimicrobial properties and so it will fight harmful bacteria and help prevent infections.

For cholesterol control coconut water is ideal as it reduces the bad cholesterol levels and increases your good cholesterol levels. Anyone who has issues with the cholesterol levels can benefit from a couple of glasses of this healing water every day. Because coconut water helps with cholesterol it means it is also good for your arteries and heart, reducing your chances of heart attack and stroke. It has also been shown to be useful for anyone recovering from myocardial damage.

A couple of glasses of coconut oil a day has also been shown to help people control high blood pressure. With a high level of antioxidants it will also help protect your liver and promote good function of it.

Coconut water is also mildly diuretic so is useful for anyone suffering from urinary problems and is great in a detox to get rid of toxins.

With high levels of antioxidants, coconut water is great at hunting down free radicals and reducing the signs of aging as well as keeping your skin and cells healthy.

Coconut water is another very beneficial part of a coconut that you can use to supplement your use of coconut oil and it can be used in some of the recipes described later in this book.

COOKING WITH COCONUT OIL

A great way to get many of the benefits of coconut oil is to cook with it. Whilst heating it will get rid of some of the nutrients there will still be plenty of left by the time you consume the meal. If you are concerned that you are not getting enough benefit from coconut oil just by cooking with it then take capsules or just eat a spoon or two of coconut oil every day.

Coconut oil is best melted in a cup placed in a bowl of warm water. Try to avoid using a microwave as this will damage the nutritional benefit of the oil.

Whilst there are a number of recipes here you can use coconut oil in almost any meal that you make by substituting the oil the recipe calls for with coconut oil. These are some of my favorite dishes that use coconut oil and you are bound to find something here you will like!

Coconut Oil Breakfasts

Coconut oil is great to include with your breakfast and there are a number of delicious breakfasts you can make which are ideal for the lazy Sunday morning or the busy day at work!

Coconut Oil Scrambled Eggs

This is a variation on the traditional scrambled eggs which uses coconut oil to fry in. It will make between three and six servings, depending on how hungry you are and take around 5 minutes to make.

Ingredients:
- 6 large eggs
- 6 teaspoons milk
- 1 tablespoon coconut oil
- Salt and pepper to taste

Method:
1. Whisk together the eggs and milk in a glass measuring bowl
2. Heat a non-stick frying pan but do not add the coconut oil yet
3. When the pan has heated add the oil
4. Once it has melted and is clear add the eggs
5. Use a wooden spoon to gently stir the eggs, ensuring they scramble and cook evening
6. Garnish with salt and pepper or even chopped fresh chives

Honey and Coconut Granola

A healthy granola that is great by itself or mixed in with a low fat yoghurt. This recipe will make enough for 10 to 12 servings and will take you around 35 minutes to make.

Ingredients:

- 5 cups cold fashioned oats
- 1 cup mixed nuts (chopped)
- ½ cup dried fruit
- ¼ cup shredded coconut
- ¼ cup flax seeds
- 1/3 cup coconut oil
- 1/3 cup honey
- 2 teaspoons ground cinnamon
- 1 teaspoon vanilla extract
- 1 teaspoon almond extract
- ½ teaspoon salt

Method:

1. Preheat your oven to 325F
2. Put the nuts, flax seed, oats, cinnamon and shredded coconut in a large bowl
3. In a separate bowl melt the coconut oil and mix in the salt, honey, vanilla extract and the almond extract
4. Pour this mixture into a baking pan
5. Bake in the middle of your oven for 15 minutes
6. Stir well then back for a further 15 minutes
7. Repeat the stirring and baking process until it reaches the desired brownness
8. Remove from the oven, stir in the dried fruit and leave to cool

Vegan Granola

This is a delicious granola that is ideal for anyone who is vegan but can be enjoyed by anyone. This recipe will make enough for 20 to 24 servings and take around 40 minutes.

Ingredients:

- 1lb raw cashew nuts (roughly chopped)
- 8oz raw almonds (sliced)
- 8oz sweetened, shaved coconut flakes
- 4oz raw hazelnuts (roughly chopped)
- 2oz sesame seeds
- 2/3 cup virgin coconut oil (melted)
- 1/3 cup pure maple syrup
- ¼ cup coconut palm sugar
- ¼ cup ground flaxseed meal
- ¼ cup almond meal
- 1 teaspoon vanilla extract
- 1 teaspoon ground cinnamon
- ½ teaspoon sea salt
- ¼ teaspoon almond extract
- Pinch of ground nutmeg

Method:

1. Position the racks in your oven at the 2nd and 4th positions from the top, preheating to 325F
2. Use a food processor to pulse the cashews and hazelnuts until they are small chunks (or chop by hand) – be careful not to powder and over process
3. In a large bowl mix together the cashews, hazelnuts, sesame seeds, flax meal, sliced almonds, palm sugar, nutmeg, cinnamon, salt, coconut meal and almond meal
4. Stir thoroughly until well combined
5. In a separate bowl mix together the melted coconut oil, maple syrup, vanilla extract and almond extract
6. Pour the wet ingredients over the dry and mix well
7. Spread the granola evenly between two baking sheets in a single layer
8. Cook for 15 minutes in the oven
9. Remove, stir and bake for a further 15 minutes swapping shelves

Pumpkin Pancakes

Pancakes make for a lovely breakfast and with coconut oil and pumpkin these are really delicious plus they are dairy free, gluten free and low in carbohydrates! This will make enough for about 12 servings.

Ingredients:

- 6 large eggs
- ½ cup coconut flour
- ½ cup pumpkin puree
- ½ cup unsweetened coconut milk (use an extra ¼ cup for a runnier batter)
- ¼ cup sweetener (substitute for honey or maple syrup if you prefer)
- ¼ cup hemp protein powder (vanilla flavored)
- 3 tablespoons coconut oil (melted)
- 1 teaspoons ground cinnamon
- 1 teaspoon baking powder
- ½ teaspoon vanilla extract
- ½ teaspoon ground ginger
- ½ teaspoon salt
- ¼ teaspoon ground cloves
- Coconut oil for frying

Method:

1. Preheat your oven to 200F
2. In a large bowl mix together the protein powder, sweetener, baking powder, coconut flour, ground ginger, ground cloves, ground cinnamon and cloves
3. In a separate bowl whisk together the pumpkin puree, coconut oil, eggs, coconut milk and vanilla extract
4. Add this wet mixture to the dry ingredients and stir thoroughly – the batter should not be too runny nor too thick so add more coconut milk a little at a time if necessary
5. Heat a large frying pan on a high heat and melt in a little coconut oil
6. Put two generous tablespoons of batter in the pan and spread to a circle 4" in diameter
7. Repeat for as many pancakes as you can fit in the pan
8. Cook until the bottom turns golden brown and the top sets around the edges
9. Flip the pancakes carefully and cook until golden brown on both sides
10. Remove from the pan and put on a plate in the oven to keep warm whilst you cook the rest of the batter

Almond Granola

Another lovely granola recipe that makes for a great breakfast or can be turned into bars to snack on during the day. This recipe will make about four cups of granola and take around quarter of an hour to make.

Ingredients:
- 3 cups old fashioned oats
- 1 cup almonds (divided)
- 1/3 cup honey
- 1/3 cup brown sugar
- 3 tablespoons coconut oil
- ½ teaspoon salt
- ¼ teaspoon vanilla extract
- 1/8 teaspoon almond extract

Method:
1. Preheat your oven to 350F
2. In your food processor blend half the almonds until they are finely chopped
3. Coarsely chop the other half
4. Put all the almonds in a large bowl and mix in with the oats, brown sugar and salt, stirring well
5. Mix together the melted coconut oil, honey, vanilla extract and almond extract
6. Pour this mixture over the oat mixture and stir well until everything is coated
7. Put the mixture on to a baking tray in a single layer
8. Bake for 5 minutes then stir and bake for a further 5 minutes
9. Cool on wax paper before storing in an airtight container

Coconut Oil Sides and Meals

Coconut oil can be used in all sorts of meals and here are some main courses, lunches and even side dishes that you can make using this miracle oil. Have fun trying these as they are absolutely delicious!

Sautéed Coconut and Ginger Shrimp

A light coconut shrimp dish with very subtle flavors that is absolutely delicious. This dish will take you about a quarter of an hour to make and will serve two.

Ingredients:
- 1lb large shrimp (shelled)
- 6 green onions (slice and reserve the green parts, slice the white parts)
- 2 garlic cloves (minced)
- 2½ tablespoons coconut oil
- 1 tablespoon fresh ginger (minced)
- 1 teaspoon fresh lemon juice
- ½ teaspoon ground coriander
- ½ teaspoon salt
- ½ teaspoon ground black pepper

Method:
1. Heat a large skillet on a medium heat and then melt the coconut oil
2. Add the white parts of the onions, reserving the green parts, together with the garlic and ginger
3. Cook, stirring constantly, for around 30 seconds until fragrant
4. Add the coriander and cook, stirring constantly, for another 30 seconds
5. Add the shrimp and salt, stirring often and cook for about 2 or 3 minutes until the shrimp turn opaque
6. Add the green parts of the onion and cook for 10 or 15 seconds until wilted
7. Season with lemon juice and pepper before serving with lemon wedges

Chorizo and Roasted Vegetable Soup

A simple soup to make that is absolutely jam packed with flavor! The roasted vegetables are tasty and soft and the chorizo creates a delightful flavor. This recipe will make ten servings and will take about an hour to cook.

Ingredients:
- 6 cups chicken or vegetable stock
- 2 cups rutabaga (cubed)
- ¼ cup coconut oil (melted and divided)
- 12oz chorizo (sliced)
- 1 medium eggplant (cubed)
- 1 medium pepper (chopped)
- 1 medium zucchini (cubed)
- 1 small onion (chopped)
- 1 teaspoon salt
- ½ teaspoon ground black pepper

Method:
1. Preheat your oven to 450F
2. In a ceramic baking dish mix together the vegetables together with the salt and pepper and coconut oil, stirring well to ensure the vegetables are well coated
3. Bake for half an hour, stirring after fifteen minutes
4. Heat a tablespoon of coconut oil in a large saucepan over a medium heat and sauté the chorizo until browned – around 8 to 10 minutes
5. Add the roasted vegetables and the stock to the saucepan and boil
6. Reduce the heat and simmer for 10 minutes before serving

Parmesan Chicken Nuggets

A very simple recipe to prepare that is surprisingly tasty. These are great to serve with a dipping sauce or with vegetables and fries.

Ingredients:

- 1lb boneless, skinless chicken breast (cut into nugget sized pieces)
- 1 egg
- 1 cup almonds
- ½ cup Parmesan cheese (grated)
- ¼ cup heavy cream
- Coconut oil for frying
- Pinch of cayenne pepper

Method:

1. Put the almonds and the cheese into your food processor and blend until they look like crumbs and are thoroughly blended
2. Using a fork whisk together the cream, egg and cayenne pepper
3. Heat an inch of oil in a pan over a medium to high heat – make sure the pan has high sides
4. Coat the chicken in the bread mixture, then the egg mixture then the bread mixture again
5. Fry in the pan on both sides until cooked through and crispy – try not to turn too many times otherwise the bread mixture comes off
6. Place on a paper towel after cooking to drain excess oil

Cauliflower Fried Rice

This is a very versatile take on an Asian classic and is easy for you to turn into a gluten free, vegan or vegetarian dish.

Ingredients:
- 1 head of cauliflower
- 7 scallions (chopped but separate the white from the dark green)
- 5 garlic cloves (chopped)
- 2 eggs (lightly beaten)
- 1lb protein of your choice (chicken, pork, shrimp, tofu, etc.)
- 4 cups cooked brown rice (cooled)
- 2 cups steamed broccoli (finely chopped)
- 1 cup steamed carrots (sliced)
- 4 tablespoons soy sauce or tamari (divided)
- 2 tablespoons coconut oil
- 1 tablespoons sesame oil
- 1 teaspoon fresh ginger (chopped)
- Optional – toasted sesame seeds or the dark green scallion tops for garnish

Method:
1. Chop the cauliflower into large florets, removing the tough stem
2. Pulse the cauliflower in your food processor until it looks like rice
3. Heat a tablespoon of coconut oil in a large skillet on a medium heat
4. Add the garlic, ginger and white parts of the scallions and sauté for two minutes until the scallions begin to soften
5. Add the cauliflower and stir well, cooking for a few more minutes until it starts to caramelize
6. Stir well then cook so it caramelizes for a few more minutes
7. Turn the heat up and add the rest of the coconut oil and the brown rice, stirring well until everything is coated
8. Flatten the mixture out in the pan and leave for a couple of minutes so the rice browns
9. Add the carrots and broccoli and stir well
10. Scoop out a well in the middle of the pan and add your protein and two tablespoons of soy sauce
11. Once this has cooked make another well and pour in the eggs, stirring rapidly to scramble them
12. Stir well then add the sesame oil and the rest of the soy sauce
13. Stir again, cook for a further 2 or 3 minutes before serving

Coconut Roasted Sweet Potatoes

Using virgin coconut oil really enhanced the sweetness of the potatoes, adding a subtle yet attractive aroma to them. This makes for a superb side dish and will make between 2 and 4 servings taking about 1 hour 10 minutes to cook.

Ingredients:
- 1¾lb sweet potatoes (peeled and diced)
- 1½ tablespoons virgin coconut oil
- 2 teaspoons light brown sugar
- ¾ teaspoon salt
- ¼ teaspoon nutmeg (freshly grated is best)
- ¼ teaspoon ground black pepper

Method:
1. Preheat your oven to 350F
2. Melt the coconut oil over a low heat in a small saucepan
3. Toss together all of the ingredients in a large bowl until the potatoes are thoroughly coated
4. Spread out in a baking pan and cook for about an hour until soft and caramelized, tossing occasionally

Coconut Chicken Patties

This is a very healthy dish that is paleo friendly. The coconut and the chicken blend together really well to give a very interesting taste. This dish will make between 4 and six servings.

Ingredients:

- 1lb ground chicken
- 1 egg yolk
- ½ cup plus 1/3 cup almond flour
- ½ cup unsweetened shredded coconut
- ½ cup coconut oil (melted)
- 1 teaspoon onion powder
- ¼ teaspoon salt
- ¼ teaspoon ground black pepper
- ¼ teaspoon garlic powder
- ¼ teaspoon paprika

Method:

1. Preheat your oven to 375F
2. In a bowl mix together the shredded coconut, ½ cup of almond flour and season well, stirring well
3. In a separate bowl mix the chicken, the rest of the almond flour together with the onion powder, paprika, egg yolk, garlic powder, salt and pepper
4. Heat a large skillet then add the coconut oil until it melts on a medium to high heat
5. Roll around two tablespoons of the chicken mixture into a ball then coat with the coconut mixture, flattening it slightly into a patty shape
6. Repeat until you have used all the mixture – it should make around 12 patties
7. Fry the patties in the coconut oil for about 3 or 4 minutes per side until golden brown
8. Once cooked place on a parchment lined baking sheet and cook in the oven for 5 to 7 minutes so the chicken is cooked through

Pistachio Pesto Pasta

This is a great recipe that is paleo diet friendly and is easy to make. This recipe will take you around 50 minutes to make and will produce 4 servings.

Ingredients:

- 4 chicken breasts (sliced or cubed depending on your preference)
- 1 spaghetti squash (halved)
- 1 cup fresh basil leaves
- 1 cup pistachio nuts (unshelled)
- ½ to 1 cup coconut oil (melted)
- 2 teaspoons fresh garlic (minced)
- 1 lemon (juiced)
- Optional toppings – chopped basil or red pepper flakes

Ingredients:

1. Preheat your oven to 425F
2. Cut the squash in half lengthwise and scoop out the seeds
3. Line a baking sheet with foil and place the squash open side down
4. Cook for between 30 and 40 minutes until the thickest part of the squash can be pierced with a fork easily
5. Put the pistachios in your food processor and process until they are finely chopped
6. Add the lemon juice, garlic and basil, seasoning with salt and pepper before grinding until it is smooth
7. Slowly pour in the coconut oil until you get the right consistency – you may not need an entire cup – then put to one side
8. Season both sides of your chicken with salt and pepper and cook (in coconut oil of course) on a medium heat until it is cooked through
9. Once the squash is cooled shred it with a fork and place it in a large serving bowl
10. Add the pesto and stir well
11. Serve either with the chicken mixed in or on top

Mahi Mahi Nuggets

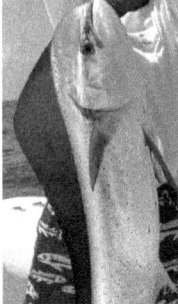

Mahi mahi or common dolphinfish is a surface dwelling dish found all over the world, typically off-shore in temperature, tropical and sub-tropical areas such as the Caribbean, Pacific Coast of the Americas, between Florida and West Africa, Southeast Asia and Hawaii. It is a popular eating fish but if you cannot get hold of it then substitute for another fish you can find.

Ingredients:
- 1¼lb mahi mahi
- 1 large egg
- 4 lime wedges
- 1 cup almond flour
- 2/3 cup unsweetened shredded coconut
- ¼ cup virgin coconut oil
- ¾ teaspoon salt
- ¼ teaspoon ground black pepper

Method:
1. Put a wire cooling rack over the top of a cookie sheet
2. Cut the fish into 1" or 2" pieces and pat dry using paper towels
3. Whisk the egg in a shallow bowl
4. In a lidded plastic container mix together the shredded coconut, almond flour, salt and pepper, shaking well to combine
5. In a large skillet on a medium heat melt 2 tablespoons of coconut oil
6. Add half the fish to the egg, tossing well to ensure it is well coated
7. Shake off excess egg and transfer using a slotted spoon to the almond flour mixture
8. Seal the container and shake until the fish is coated
9. Cook in your heated skillet for between 2 and 4 minutes per side until the crust turns a light golden brown color
10. Transfer the cooked fish to the cooling rack (keep warm in the oven if you want)
11. Repeat the process for the rest of the fish and serve with lime wedges

Thai Fish Cakes

This gluten free, low carb dish makes a fantastic appetizer, serving 5 or 6, or a delicious main course, serving 3 or 4. This recipe uses a fish called Barramundi which is a very nice white fish with firm flesh. Substitute this for an alternative white, firm fleshed fish if necessary.

Ingredients:
- 1lb barramundi fillets (remove the skin and cut into 1" cubes)
- 2 garlic cloves
- 3 tablespoons fish sauce
- 3 tablespoons coconut butter
- 2 tablespoons coconut oil
- 1 tablespoon fresh cilantro leaves
- 1 tablespoons fresh ginger (grated)
- ½ teaspoon chilli powder
- ½ teaspoon red pepper flakes
- ½ teaspoon ground cumin
- ¼ teaspoon ground coriander
- Garnish – lime wedges

Spicy Mayo Ingredients:
- 3 tablespoons mayonnaise
- ½ to 1 teaspoon of hot sauce

Method:
1. The mayo is made by mixing the hot sauce and mayonnaise in a small bowl, then putting to one side
2. Put the rest of the ingredients in to your food blender, except the coconut oil
3. Pulse until you have a thick paste, scraping the sides of the mixer bowl as required
4. Shape into 1½" inch balls and press down into patty shapes that are about ¾" thick (wet your hands to prevent the mixture sticking to you)
5. Heat a tablespoon of coconut oil in a large skillet on a medium heat
6. Cook the fish cakes for 1 to 2 minutes per side until golden brown in color and cooked throughout
7. Remove from the oil and put on paper towels whilst you cook the rest of the fish cakes
8. Serve with a spot of the spicy mayo and garnished with lime wedges

Paleo Chicken Curry

This is a fantastic curry and the coconut really enhances the taste, giving you the benefit not only of coconut oil but also of the coconut milk itself. It is great when served with jasmine or basmati rice and can be served topped with some shredded coconut. This recipe will make enough for about 8 servings and take about half an hour to make.

Ingredients:

- 8 boneless and skinless chicken thighs (cut into 1" cubes)
- 3 small zucchini (cut in half lengthwise and slice thickly)
- 1 large onion (cut into large chunks)
- 30oz coconut milk
- 1 cup grape tomatoes (yellow or red)
- 2 tablespoons coconut oil
- 1 tablespoon curry powder
- 2 teaspoons coarse salt
- 1 teaspoon garlic (minced)
- ½ teaspoon paprika
- Chopped cilantro or shredded coconut to garnish

Method:

1. Melt the coconut oil in a large saucepan over a medium to high heat
2. Cook the chicken until it is browned on both sides and cooked through
3. Remove the chicken from the pan and put to one side, leaving the oil in the pan
4. Add the zucchini and onion and sauté until lightly browned
5. Add the paprika, salt, curry powder and garlic, cooking for a further 30 seconds stirring constantly
6. Return the chicken to the pan and add the coconut oil
7. Bring the pan to the boil before reducing the heat, covering and simmering for about half an hour until the chicken is tender
8. 5 minutes before the dish is ready add the tomatoes and stir them in

Coconut Curry Crockpot

Crockpots are a great way for you to cook meals and I am a big fan of them! This is a delicious curry that has a very subtle coconut flavor making it ideal for anyone who doesn't like a curry that is too strong. This recipe will serve four people and take about three and a half hours to cook.

Ingredients:
- 14½oz container of seafood stock
- 20 medium shrimp (peeled)
- 2 celery stalks (chopped)
- 1 small onion (chopped)
- 1 garlic clove (minced)
- 1 sweet potato (chopped)
- 1 cup tofu (drained and chopped)
- ¼ cup coconut cream
- 2 teaspoons curry powder (any strength you like)
- 1 teaspoon lemon juice

Method:
1. Add everything into your crockpot and stir well
2. Cook for about 3 hours on the high setting or until the potatoes are tender

Coconut Hollandaise Sauce

This is a great sauce that is dairy free and also paleo diet friendly. It is slightly thinner in consistency than the sauce made with butter but is still absolutely delicious. Any extra sauce can be kept in your refrigerator and used the next day, just heat it on a low heat for a few minutes. It will take you about 15 minutes to prepare and cook this recipe. It is great with eggs benedict, salmon or asparagus.

Ingredients:

- 2 medium egg yolks
- 3 tablespoons coconut oil (melted)
- 1 tablespoon lemon juice
- ½ teaspoon salt
- 1/8 teaspoon paprika

Method:

1. Fill your blender with boiling water, cover and leave to stand for 10 minutes
2. Empty the water out then dry the blender
3. Add the egg yolks and lemon juice and blend thoroughly
4. With the blender on a low speed slowly pour in the melted coconut oil
5. Add the salt and pepper and pulse a few more times until well combined

Garlic and Rosemary Roast Beef

This is a fantastic Sunday roast or family meal that is absolutely delicious. If you can find grass fed beef then it is better as it is paleo diet friendly plus it has a much richer taste than normal beef.

Ingredients:
- 3lb beef joint
- 15 to 20 garlic cloves (turn into a paste in your food processor)
- 3 sprigs fresh rosemary
- ½ cup coconut oil (melted)
- Vegetables of choice (chopped into bite sized pieces – potatoes, carrots, sweet potatoes, rutabaga, swede, parsnip all work well here)

Method:
1. The day before you cook the roast mix the garlic cloves and rosemary leaves into a paste (use a blender)
2. Rub this mixture over the outside of the roast, turning to ensure it is thoroughly covered
3. Season generously, cover and refrigerate overnight
4. Remove the roast from the refrigerator about half an hour to an hour before cooking to allow it to warm to room temperature
5. Preheat your oven to 400F
6. Chop the vegetables and put them in your roasting pan with your roast – use any vegetables you like but remember that harder vegetables will take longer to soften so you may need to cut vegetables like carrots and parsnips into smaller chunks than say a sweet potato so all the vegetables are ready at the same time
7. Drizzle the melted coconut oil over the vegetables and season well
8. Cook the roast, uncovered, for 15 minutes before reducing the heat to 300F
9. Cook for between 60 and 75 minutes before temperature testing to ensure it is cooked – as a guide a temperature of 120F is rare, 130F is medium rare, 140F is medium, 150F is medium to well done and over 160F is well done
10. Remember that the beef will continue to cook when removed from the oven so remove it when it reaches the desired temperature, cover and allow it to stand for about 10 minutes
11. Slice and serve with a home-made gravy

Chicken and Vegetable Curry

Another simple curry recipe that is easy to make and thoroughly delightful. Coconut lends itself well to Indian and Asian dishes and this can be served topped with shredded coconut. This recipe produces enough to serve between 4 and 6 and can be served with jasmine or basmati rice.

Ingredients:
- 24oz strained tomatoes (passata) or tomato sauce
- 4 carrots (chopped)
- 2 garlic cloves (minced)
- 2 poblano peppers (chopped)
- 1 zucchini (chopped)
- 1 onion (chopped)
- 1 yellow squash (chopped)
- 1 can coconut milk (full fat works best)
- 1lb chicken (shredded, sliced or cubed)
- 1 cup chopped parsley
- 1 cup chopped cilantro
- 2 to 4 tablespoons coconut oil
- 2 tablespoons curry powder
- ¾ teaspoon salt

Method:
1. In a large frying pan melt 2 tablespoons of coconut oil on a medium to high heat
2. Brown the chicken then add the garlic, onion, carrots and peppers
3. Cook for 5 minutes before adding the zucchini and squash, stirring well – if it starts to stick then use more coconut oil
4. Reduce the heat to a medium low heat and add the coconut milk, curry powder, salt and strained tomatoes
5. Cover and allow to simmer before reducing the heat to low and leaving to simmer for 20 to 30 minutes until the vegetables are tender
6. About five minutes before serving stir in the cilantro and parsley
7. Test for flavor, adding more salt or curry powder if necessary before serving

Jerk Chicken

This is a spicy island chicken that will surprise you with the depth of flavor. It is served on a bed of brown rice and will take about an hour and a half to make, serving six people.

Ingredients:
- 2lb skinless, bones chicken breast (cubed)
- 28oz can chopped peeled tomatoes (reserve the juice)
- 13½oz can coconut milk
- 8oz button mushrooms (sliced)
- 1 onion (coarsely chopped)
- 1 bunch green onions (sliced)
- 1 cup butternut squash (peeled, seeded and diced)
- ½ cup tomato juice
- 2 tablespoons coconut oil
- 1 tablespoon white sugar
- 2 teaspoons chicken bouillon granules
- 2 teaspoons curry powder
- 2 teaspoons dry Caribbean jerk seasoning
- 1 teaspoon fresh garlic (minced)

Method:
1. Melt the coconut oil in a skillet on a medium heat then stir in the onions, garlic, curry powder, bouillon granules and jerk seasoning
2. Stir well and cook for a couple of minutes
3. Reduce the heat slightly then add the chicken
4. Cook for a further 6 to 8 minutes, stirring often
5. Add the mushrooms, squash and all put a tablespoon of the green onion (which is reserved for garnish) and stir well, cooking for an additional 2 minutes
6. Add the tomatoes, ½ cup of tomato juice, coconut milk and sugar
7. Stir well, reduce the heat and simmer for 35 to 40 minutes, stirring occasionally
8. Serve hot on a bed of rice garnished with green onion

Tofu Mango Tacos

This is a very interesting vegetarian Mexican dish that is surprisingly tasty. Of course you can use beans or meat if you want but this dish stands well by itself. Red taco sauces tend to work best with this dish and any extra filling can either be heated up later on used as salsa!

Ingredients:

- 2 x 14oz tofu packages (cut into chunks)
- ½ packet of red taco seasoning mix (divided)
- 2 mangos (peeled and cubed)
- 2 garlic cloves (finely chopped)
- 1 onion (chopped)
- 1 chilli pepper of your choice (chopped)
- Bunch of fresh cilantro (finely chopped – separate the leaves and stems)
- 3 tablespoons coconut oil
- 1 teaspoon ground coriander
- 1 teaspoon ground cumin
- Pinch of chilli powder
- Salt to taste

Method:

1. Heat the coconut oil in a skillet on a medium heat
2. Sauté the onion, garlic and pepper for about ten minutes until the onion is lightly browned
3. Add the tofu and stir well until it is coated
4. Stir in the cilantro stems, ¼ packet of taco seasoning plus a teaspoon each of cumin and ground coriander
5. Cook for about 5 minutes, stirring often until fragrant and the tofu is cooked throughout
6. Add the mango plus another ¼ packet of taco seasoning and leave for 4 or 5 minutes before stirring
7. Add the salt and chilli powder, stirring to coat and season with more coriander and cumin if desired
8. Simmer for about 10 minutes until most of the liquid has evaporated
9. Stir in the chopped cilantro leaves about a minute before serving

Coconut Oil Desserts and Sweet Treats

Coconuts have a delicious sweet flavor that makes it ideal for any dessert. Here you will learn some great sweet coconut recipes that can be eaten as desserts or as a sweet treat for you during the day.

Rice Krispie Treats

When made with coconut oil these treats are surprisingly delicious! This recipe takes about 15 minutes to prepare.

Ingredients:
- 10oz mini marshmallows
- 5 cups crispy rice cereal
- 2 tablespoons coconut oil
- 2 tablespoons butter

Method:
1. Melt the coconut oil and butter in a large saucepan on a low to medium heat
2. Add the marshmallows and stir until they start to melt
3. Remove from the heat and stir in the cereal, ensuring it is evenly mixed
4. Grease a 8x8" pan and put the mixture into it, flattening down the top
5. Leave for about an hour to cool then cut and enjoy

Banana Walnut Bread

A very interesting bread that makes great use of ripe bananas plus as it uses whole wheat flour it is healthier for you. With the coconut oil and agave nectar it has a much lower glycemic index and so is much healthier for you. It will take about an hour to make this bread.

Ingredients:

- 4 ripe bananas (mashed)
- 2 cups whole wheat flour
- 2/3 cup agave nectar
- ½ cup walnuts (chopped – for the bread)
- 1/3 cup coconut oil (melted)
- 1/3 cup walnuts (chopped – for the topping)
- 1 egg
- 2 tablespoons sour cream
- 1 teaspoon baking soda
- ½ teaspoon vanilla extract
- ¼ teaspoon salt

Method:

1. Preheat your oven to 325F and great a 9x5x3" loaf pan, dusting it with flour
2. In a large mixing bowl combine the dry ingredients, ensuring they are well mixed
3. Mash together the bananas and the wet ingredients to form a paste
4. Add the wet ingredients to the dry ingredients and stir together
5. Add ½ cup walnuts and stir
6. Pour the mixture into your loaf pan and top with the rest of the walnuts
7. Bake for between 45 and 60 minutes until a toothpick inserted into the middle of the bread comes out clean

Pumpkin Muffins

Pumpkin is an underused ingredient that is absolutely delicious and makes for some fantastic recipes. These muffins make use of canned pumpkin though you can use pureed fresh pumpkin if you prefer. It takes about 35 minutes to complete this recipe.

Ingredients:
- 2 large eggs
- 7½oz can of pureed pumpkin
- 1 1/3 cups whole wheat pastry flour
- 2/3 cups sugar
- 4 tablespoons coconut oil
- ½ teaspoon ground cinnamon
- ½ teaspoon pumpkin pie spice
- ½ teaspoon vanilla extract
- ¼ teaspoon salt
- Optional – sliced almonds for topping

Method:
1. Preheat your oven to 375F and line your muffin tray with 6 paper liners
2. Beat together the sugar and melted coconut oil using an electric mixer
3. Add the pumpkin, vanilla and eggs and beat until the mixture is smooth
4. In a separate bowl mix together the baking powder, spices, salt and flour
5. Blend this into the pumpkin mixture
6. Divide this batter between the muffin cups (it should come close to the top)
7. Decorate with sliced almonds
8. Bake for 22 to 25 minutes until a toothpick inserted into the middle of a muffin comes out clean

Lemon and Blueberry Muffins

Another fantastic muffin recipe with some really interesting flavors. This recipe contains a natural sweetener that makes it healthier than many other muffin recipes.

Ingredients:
- 2½ cups all-purpose flour
- 1½ cups fresh blueberries (washed and dried)
- 1 cup milk
- ¾ cup Stevia (plus some extra to sprinkle on the top of the muffins)
- ½ coconut oil (melted)
- 2 large eggs
- 1 tablespoon baking powder
- 1 tablespoon freshly grated lemon zest
- 1 teaspoon lemon juice
- 1 teaspoon ground nutmeg
- ½ teaspoon vanilla extract
- Pinch of sea salt

Method:
1. Preheat your oven to 425F and line your muffin tin with 12 paper liners
2. In a medium sized bowl whisk together the Stevia, baking powder, nutmeg, salt and flour
3. In a separate bowl mix together the eggs, lemon zest, lemon juice, vanilla extract, milk and coconut oil
4. Slowly pour the wet ingredients into the dry, stirring well until there are no lumps and the mixture is thoroughly combined
5. Mix in the blueberries
6. Divide the batter evenly between the liners and sprinkle the tops with Stevia
7. Put the muffins into your oven and turn the temperature down to 375F
8. Bake until golden brown, about 25 minutes, turning the muffin tin at the halfway point
9. You know they are ready when a toothpick pushed into the middle of a muffin comes out clean
10. Cool in a wire rack for 10 minutes before enjoying

Cinnamon Cookies

These are lovely cookies, simple to make, taking about 20 minutes and easy to eat!

Ingredients:

- 1 large egg
- 1½ cups all-purpose flour
- 1 cup brown sugar
- ½ cup coconut oil (melted)
- 1½ teaspoons vanilla extract
- 1½ teaspoons ground cinnamon
- ¾ teaspoon baking powder
- ½ teaspoon baking soda
- Pinch of salt

Method:

1. Preheat your oven to 350F and line two cookie sheets with parchment paper
2. In a medium bowl mix together the baking powder, baking soda, cinnamon, flour and salt
3. In a stand mixer mix together the brown sugar and coconut oil until fluffy
4. Beat in the vanilla extract and egg
5. Slowly add the wet ingredients to the dry, stirring until well combined
6. Use a cookie scooper to scoop the dough onto the baking sheets
7. Cook for 9 to 11 minutes
8. Remove from the oven and leave to cool for 4 or 5 minutes before transferring to a wire rack to cool

Nutty Banana Scones

This is a nice vegan recipe that makes some delicious scones which, if you want to be truly decadent and non-vegan, can be served with traditional Cornish clotted cream and Strawberry jam.

Ingredients:
- 2 cups whole wheat flour
- 1 cup raw pecans
- ¾ cup ripe banana (mashed)
- 1/3 cup coconut oil
- ¼ cup milk (can use normal milk, soy or almond milk)
- 2 tablespoons maple syrup (you can use honey instead)
- 1 tablespoon baking powder
- 1 teaspoon ground cinnamon
- ½ teaspoon vanilla extract
- ½ teaspoon ground ginger
- ½ teaspoon salt

Maple Glaze Ingredients:
- 1 cup powdered sugar
- ¼ cup maple syrup
- 1 tablespoon coconut oil (melted)
- ½ teaspoon vanilla extract
- 1/8 teaspoon sea salt

Method:
1. Preheat your oven to 425F
2. Line a rimmed baking sheet with parchment paper and place the nuts in a single layer on it
3. Bake for about 3 minutes then finely chop the nuts
4. In a medium sized mixing bowl mi together the flour, ¾ of the nuts, baking powder, ginger, cinnamon and salt ensuring it is well combined
5. Cut the coconut oil into the dry ingredients using a pastry cutter or a fork
6. Mix together the banana, ¼ cup of milk, maple syrup and vanilla extract until well combined
7. Power this into the dry mixture and stir well – it will take a little while to mix properly
8. Turn the dough out onto a flat surface and make it into a circle shape about an inch thick
9. Cut this into 8 slices

10. Place the slices on a parchment paper lined baking sheet and cook for 15 minutes until a light golden brown color
11. Whisk together the glaze ingredients until smooth (warming the coconut oil if necessary)
12. Allow the scones to cool for a few minutes before drizzling the glaze over the scones and sprinkling with the rest of the chopped nuts

Choco-Raisin Cookies

These are very nice cookies that are paleo diet friendly, containing none of the traditional ingredients. It will take about half an hour to make these 24 small, but delicious, cookies.

Ingredients:

- 1 ripe banana
- 2 1/3 cups oats
- 2/3 cup applesauce (unsweetened)
- 2/3 cup almond meal
- ½ cup raisins
- ½ cup chocolate chips
- 1/3 cup honey
- ¼ cup coconut oil
- 1 teaspoon baking powder
- 1 teaspoon vanilla extract
- ½ teaspoon ground cinnamon
- ½ teaspoon salt

Method:

1. Preheat your oven to 350F
2. Using a mix, mix together the honey, coconut oil (melted if necessary), vanilla extract, banana and applesauce
3. Add in the salt, baking powder, oats, ground cinnamon and almond meal and stir until well combined
4. Stir in the raisins and chocolate chips, ensuring they are evenly distributed
5. Place tablespoon sized lumps of the dough on to a baking sheet lined with parchment paper
6. Bake for 10 to 12 minutes until you can start smelling the cookies
7. Remove from the oven and cool on wire racks

Banana and Walnut Muffins

Another great muffin recipe which makes for a great snack, dessert or even a breakfast if you prefer!

Ingredients:

- 2 ripe bananas (mashed)
- 1 egg
- 2/3 cup whole wheat flour
- ½ cup quick cooking oats
- ½ cup almond milk (unsweetened)
- ½ cup walnuts (chopped)
- ¼ cup Stevia
- 2 tablespoons coconut oil (melted)
- 1¾ teaspoons baking powder
- ¾ teaspoon vanilla extract
- ½ teaspoon cinnamon
- ¼ teaspoon salt

Method:

1. Preheat your oven to 350F and line a muffin tin with paper liners
2. In a medium sized bowl mix together the almond milk, egg, coconut oil, vanilla extract and banana until thoroughly combined and put to one side
3. In a separate bowl mix together the oats, flour, Stevia, cinnamon, salt, walnuts and baking powder
4. Stir the flour mixture into the banana mixture until it is well combined
5. Divide the batter evenly between the muffin cups
6. Bake for 20 to 25 minutes until a toothpick inserted into the middle comes out clean
7. Decorate with chopped walnuts, cool and enjoy

Coconut Donuts

A low carb donut recipe that has a really coconut flavor and is grain and gluten free! This recipe will make about ten medium sized donuts and take 20-25 minutes to make.

Ingredients:
- 4 large eggs
- ½ cup coconut flour
- ½ cup almond milk (unsweetened)
- ¼ cup sweetener of your choice (Stevia is my favorite)
- ¼ cup coconut oil (melted)
- 1 teaspoon baking powder
- ½ teaspoon vanilla extract
- ¼ teaspoon Stevia
- ¼ teaspoon salt
- Coconut oil for frying

Coating Ingredients:
- ¼ cup shredded coconut (lightly toasted)
- ¼ cup powdered sweetener

Method:
1. Preheat your oven to 325F and grease a donut pan
2. In a large bowl mix together the sweetener, baking powder, salt and coconut flour
3. Stir in the coconut oil, almond milk, Stevia, vanilla extract and eggs until well combined
4. Fill the wells in the donut pan until they are about 2/3 full
5. Bake for about 15 minutes until set and just starting to turn brown around the edges
6. Remove from the oven and leave in the pan for 5 minutes before turning out onto a wire rack to cool
7. Repeat with any remaining batter
8. In a large skillet melt coconut oil until it is about ½" deep over a medium heat
9. Mix together the coating ingredients into a shallow bowl
10. Add 4 or 5 donuts to the pan and fry for a minute or two on both sides (they will brown quickly)
11. Remove the donuts from the pan and press down both sides in the coating
12. Cool for a couple of minutes on a wire rack and then eat warm!

Raspberry Scones

Another great scone recipe though feel free to replace the raspberries with any other fruit you like.

Ingredients:

- 2½ cups almond flour
- 1 cup frozen raspberries
- ½ cup shredded coconut (unsweetened)
- ½ cup golden flax seed meal
- ½ cup powdered sweetener
- 1/3 cup coconut oil (melted)
- ¼ cup almond milk
- 2 large eggs (beaten lightly)
- 1 tablespoon baking powder
- ½ teaspoon vanilla extract
- ¼ teaspoon salt

Method:

1. Preheat your oven to 325F and line a cookie sheet with parchment paper
2. In a large bowl combine the sweetener, salt, baking powder, shredded coconut, almond flour and flax seed meal
3. Stir in the eggs, almond milk, vanilla extract and coconut oil to make a sticky dough
4. Stir in the raspberries until they are evenly distributed
5. Turn the dough out onto the cookie sheet and shape into a 6x8" rectangle
6. Cut into 6 then cut each part in half diagonally to make a triangular shape
7. Separate the scones and spread out on the cookie sheet, leaving an inch between them
8. Bake for 28 to 30 minutes until firm to the touch and golden brown

Whole Wheat Waffles

These are a healthy waffle that makes for a great dessert and can be heated up for a breakfast. This will make thin waffles though you can make them into thicker Belgian style waffles. Top with maple syrup, bananas or anything else you fancy! It only takes about 15 minutes to make these waffles and they can be frozen and heated in a toaster

Ingredients:
- 1 large egg (beaten)
- 1½ cups whole wheat flour
- 1½ cups milk
- 1/3 cup virgin coconut oil (melted)
- 2 tablespoons white sugar
- 2 teaspoons baking powder
- ½ teaspoon vanilla extract
- ½ teaspoon salt

Method:
1. Preheat your waffle iron
2. In a bowl whisk together the sugar, flour, salt and baking powder
3. Make a well in the middle of this mixture
4. In a separate bowl beat together the egg, coconut oil, vanilla extract and milk
5. Pour this into the well in the dry ingredients and stir until the batter is just combined
6. Put the batter in to your waffle iron (follow the instructions) and cook for between 2 and 5 minutes until crisp and golden

Cornbread

A great cornbread that is healthy and will help to improve your good cholesterol levels. It takes about 50 minutes to make this loaf.

Ingredients:

- 2½ cups milk
- 2 cups all-purpose flour
- 1½ cups cornmeal
- ½ cup coconut oil (melted)
- ½ cup white sugar
- 2 eggs (beaten)
- 1½ tablespoons baking powder
- 1 teaspoon salt

Method:

1. Preheat your oven to 400F and grease a 9x13" baking dish or loaf tin
2. Stir together the milk and cornmeal so the cornmeal is wet all over and leave to soak for 5 minutes
3. In a separate bowl mix together the sugar, baking powder, sale and flour
4. Add in the cornmeal mixture, coconut oil and eggs, stirring until it is smooth
5. Pour this batter into your baking dish
6. Bake for 30 to 35 minutes until a toothpick pushed into the middle comes out clean

Cranberry and Ginger Snack Bars

These are excellent snack bars for anyone on the go and are really easy to make, taking just 45 minutes!

Ingredients:

- 3 cups cranberries (fresh or frozen)
- 2 cups raisins or sultanas or a mix of the two
- 1 cup water
- ¼ cup fresh ginger (grated)
- 2 apples (cored and finely chopped)

Base and Topping Ingredients:

- 2 cups brown rice flour
- 2 cups rolled oats
- ½ cup rice syrup
- ¾ cup raw sunflower seeds
- ¼ cup potato flour
- 2/3 cup coconut oil
- 1 teaspoon liquid Stevia (dissolved in 3 tablespoons water)
- ½ teaspoon salt

Method:

1. Preheat your oven to 350F and grease a 9x13" baking pan (rimmed ideally)
2. Mix the dry ingredients together in a large bowl
3. In a separate bowl mix together the oil, stevia and rice syrup
4. Combine the two sets of ingredients and mix well
5. Put 1½ cups of the crumb mixture to one side to use as a topping
6. Press the rest of the mixture into your baking pan
7. Mix together the cranberry ingredients and spread over the top of this
8. Sprinkle with the rest of the crumbs
9. Bake for about 35 minutes

Choco-Coco Bar

A wonderful bar that combines the best of chocolate with the delights of coconut complete with healthy fats! This is a great, healthy sweet treat plus it is vegan!

Ingredients:

- ½ cup cocoa
- 1/3 cup raisins
- ¼ cup coconut palm sugar (finely ground)
- ¼ cup coconut oil (melted)
- 2 tablespoons almond milk
- 1 tablespoon shredded coconut plus extra for sprinkling
- ¼ teaspoon vanilla extract
- ¼ teaspoon liquid Stevia

Method:

1. Grease an 8" square pan
2. Mix the coconut oil, coconut sugar and Stevia together
3. Add the cocoa and stir well
4. Add the almond milk a tablespoon at a time, stirring well
5. Mix in the shredded coconut and raisins
6. Spread the mixture evenly in your pan and sprinkle with coconut
7. Leave in your refrigerator to set or put in your freezer for a quicker result
8. Cut into squares and serve

Chocolate Chip Muffins

These are paleo diet friendly, easy to make and will make about 12 delicious mini muffins!

Ingredients:

- ¾ cup almond flour
- 1 egg
- 2 tablespoons virgin coconut oil (melted)
- 2 tablespoons honey or maple syrup
- 2 tablespoons mini chocolate chips
- ½ teaspoon vanilla extract
- ¼ teaspoon baking soda
- Pinch of sea salt

Method:

1. Preheat your oven to 350F, put the rack in the middle and grease a mini muffin tin
2. In a bowl mix together the baking soda, salt and almond flour
3. Add in the butter, honey, vanilla extract and egg and stir until it is just combined
4. Carefully fold in the chocolate chips
5. Fill the muffin tins ¾ full with the mixture
6. Bake for 8 or 9 minutes until a toothpick inserted into the middle of a muffin comes out clean
7. Remove from the oven, leave to cool in the pan for a couple of minutes before turning out on to a wire rack

Orange and Blueberry Scones

Paleo diet friendly scones that are gluten free, making them ideal for a snack or breakfast! It takes about 25 minutes to prepare these eight scones.

Ingredients:

- 1½ cup almond milk (or whole milk)
- 1 cup coconut flour
- 1 cup cashew flour
- 1 cup almond flour
- ½ cup blueberries (frozen)
- ¼ cup coconut sugar
- 1 tablespoon coconut oil
- 2 teaspoons baking powder
- Zest of 1 orange
- Pinch of salt

Method:

1. Preheat your oven to 400F and line a baking sheet with parchment paper
2. In a large bowl mix together the baking powder, salt and flours until thoroughly combined
3. Cut in the coconut oil whilst it is hard using a fork or your hands until it is evenly dispersed and the mixture has taken on a crumbly, pastry type appearance
4. Mix in the orange zest and sugar
5. Add the milk and stir well
6. Carefully fold in the blueberries until they are evenly dispersed
7. Put the dough on the baking sheet and spread it out into a 10-12" circle that is 1"thick
8. Optionally you can sprinkle the dough with sugar at this point and gently push it in
9. Cut the dough into 8 evenly sized pieces
10. Bake for 18 to 22 minutes until the edges start to brown and become crispy
11. Remove from the oven and leave to cool for 10 minutes on the baking sheet before separating and turning out onto a wire rack to finish cooling

Choco-Raspberry Chip Muffins

Another fantastic muffin recipe that is gluten free and low in carbs. It is an ideal breakfast or a great healthy snack for hungry children. This recipe will make 12 muffins and take about 35 minutes to make.

Ingredients:
- 3oz dark chocolate chips
- 6 large eggs
- 1 cup raspberries (frozen)
- ¾ cup powdered sweetener
- ½ cup coconut flour
- ½ cup shredded coconut (unsweetened)
- ½ cup almond milk (can be substituted with water)
- 1/3 cup coconut oil (melted)
- 1 tablespoon baking powder
- 1 teaspoon vanilla extract
- ¼ teaspoon salt

Method:
1. Preheat your oven to 350F and line your muffin pan with paper liners
2. Mix together the coconut flour, sweetener, salt, baking powder and shredded coconut in a large bowl until well combined
3. Stir in the coconut oil, eggs, vanilla extract and almond milk
4. Finally stir in the chocolate chips and raspberries
5. Divide the batter between the muffin cups
6. Bake for 20 minutes until lightly browned and firm to touch (do the toothpick test if you need to)
7. Remove from the oven and cool for 15 minutes before eating

Chocolate Candies

This is a very simple recipe for making chocolate candies that are really tasty. Make them big or small depending on how you want to control your calorie intake. These take just ten minutes to make plus half hour cooling time!

Ingredients:

- ½ cup coconut oil
- ¼ cup cocoa powder
- 2 tablespoons honey
- 1 teaspoon vanilla extract

Method:

1. Melt the coconut oil and honey together
2. Whisk up and then add the cocoa powder and vanilla extract
3. Pour into a silicone ice cube mold and cool for half an hour in your fridge or freezer

Chocolate Peanut Butter Balls

These are a really delicious treat and you may struggle to make enough of these as they are so good! This recipe makes 10 balls and takes about 25 minutes to complete. If you find that your chocolate does not harden properly then put the balls in the freezer for 10 or 15 minutes until it does harden.

Peanut Butter Ingredients:
- 1 cup confectioners' sugar
- 11 tablespoons peanut butter
- 3 tablespoons butter (softened)

Shell Ingredients:
- 6 tablespoons semi-sweet chocolate chips
- 3 tablespoons coconut oil

Method:
1. Mix together the peanut butter ingredients in a bowl until well combined
2. Shape this into 1" balls and place on a parchment paper lined baking sheet
3. Place in your freezer whilst you prepare the shell
4. Using a double boiler, melt the coconut oil and chocolate chips together, stirring often and scraping the sides
5. It will take about 5 minutes to become smooth
6. Remove from the heat and put the chocolate to one side for 5 minutes
7. Dip each peanut butter oil in the melted chocolate until it is evenly coated
8. Place the coated balls back on the baking sheet
9. Refrigerate or freeze for 10 to 20 minutes.

COCONUT OIL DRINKS

Whilst you can cook with coconut oil you can also drink it too. The only issue with putting this oil in drinks is it can clump in cold drinks and float on the top of hot drinks, which come people find off putting.

With cold drinks it is best to blend the coconut oil into a thick drink like a milkshake or smoothie. With thinner cold drinks you will end up with clumps or emulsion on the top of the drink.

For a hot drink you can whisk in the coconut oil or even mix it with honey to help delay it floating to the top. If you are bothered by this then just stir it back in to your drink before taking a sip. With a drink like hot chocolate, mix the coconut oil in with the dry ingredients which will help prevent problems.

Here are some of my favorite coconut oil drinks, all of which are pretty easy to make and are great to drink. Of course, they have many more health benefits than just the coconut oil!

Avocado Shake

This is a very creamy milkshake that can be made with cow's milk or alternatively use coconut milk or almond milk if you prefer. It only takes a few minutes to make and will serve two.

Ingredients:
- 1 avocado
- 1½ cups milk
- 2 tablespoons raw honey
- 1 to 4 tablespoons coconut oil (melted)
- ½ teaspoon vanilla extract
- 5 ice cubes

Method:
1. Remove the stone and scoop out all of the avocado flesh
2. Place this and everything else (though not the coconut oil) into your blender and blender
3. Slowly pour in the coconut oil whilst blending and serve

Lemon Green Tea

Green tea is known to be high in anti-oxidants and to be really good for you. This sweetened tea is fantastic and combines the health benefits of lemon and coconut oil too. This makes a single serving and will take a few minutes to prepare.

Ingredients:
- 1 green tea bag
- ½ fresh lemon
- 1-3 teaspoons coconut oil
- 1 teaspoon raw honey (optional)

Method:
1. Heat the water to 175F (just before it boils)
2. In a mug mix together the honey and coconut oil
3. Place the teabag into the mug
4. Squeeze the lemon juice in too
5. Pour in the hot water and leave to steep for a couple of minutes until the desired strength is reached

Morning Detox Drink

This is a fantastic drink to have first thing in the morning instead of coffee. The combination of ingredients help you to stay hydrated, detox, improve your digestion and boost your energy levels for the day. The lemon and coconut oil helps to improve the function of your kidneys and draw toxins out of your body, leaving your healthier and feeling better. After a few days of drinking this in the morning you will really be able to notice the difference.

This is very easy to make, just squeeze the juice of half a lemon into a mug together with a tablespoon of coconut oil and fill with hot water. Stir until dissolved and then drink.

Coconut Coffee

A lovely coffee drink which is surprisingly sweet as well as good for you! Coffee itself is high in anti-oxidants and so combined with the coconut oil it really gives your body a chance at fighting aging free radicals.

Ingredients:
1 cup hot coffee
1 tablespoon coconut oil
1 tablespoon unsalted butter

Method:
Put the ingredients into your blender and mix until the butter has melted and the drink is frothy!

Spinach and Apricot Smoothie

A great smoothie that is packed full of goodness to energy you and give you a great vitamin shot.

Ingredients:
- 2 cups spinach
- 1 apricot
- 1 cup coconut water
- ½ tablespoon coconut oil

Method:
1. Blend all the ingredients in your blender until they reach to desired consistency

Cocoa Smoothie

Another fantastic smoothie that is not only delicious but jam packed with super foods. It is great for breakfast, for dessert or just for an energy boost during the day.

Ingredients:
- 1 cup kale (chopped)
- ½ cup fresh strawberries (chopped)
- ½ cup fresh blueberries
- ½ to ¾ cup cooled, brewed green tea
- 1/8 cup oats
- 1/8 cup unsweetened cocoa
- 1 tablespoon honey
- 1 tablespoon chia seeds
- 1 tablespoon coconut oil

Method:
1. Place all the ingredients into your blender and blend until smooth!
2. Adjust the consistency by changing the amount of green tea to make it thicker or thinner

Green Goddess

Another great smoothie that is full of vitamins and minerals which will give your body a much needed boost.

Ingredients:
- 1 banana (frozen and broken into chunks)
- 1 kiwi (peeled)
- ¾ cup of either water, apple juice or a non-dairy milk
- Handful of kale (remove the stems)
- 1 tablespoon spirulina powder
- 1 teaspoon coconut oil

Method:
1. Blend all the ingredients together until smooth

Apple and Raspberry Smoothie
A thick, tasty smoothie that has a lot of vitamins and minerals in it. This is a fantastic smoothie for when you are run down or after a workout when you need a boost.

Ingredients:
- 1 cup ice cubes
- ½ cup plain Greek yogurt
- 1/3 cup frozen raspberries
- 1 apple (cored and coarsely chopped)
- 3 tablespoons golden raisins
- 2 tablespoons old fashioned oats
- 1 tablespoon coconut oil
- 1 tablespoon ground flax seed
- 1 tablespoons frozen apple juice concentrate
- ¼ teaspoon ground cinnamon
- ¼ teaspoon freshly grated nutmeg
- 1/8 teaspoon almond extract
- 1/8 teaspoon chia seeds to garnish

Method:
2. Microwave the raisins and apple juice concentrate in a bowl for about 30 seconds
3. Stir in the coconut oil and leave to one side
4. Blend together everything except the ice cubes until smooth, including the raisin mixture
5. Add the ice cubes a couple at a time until you reach the desired consistency
6. Divide between two glasses and top with chia seeds

Mango and Coconut Smoothie

A tropical beach in a glass! This is a delicious smoothie that makes enough for one and tastes divine.

Ingredients:

- 1 mango (peeled, de-stoned and sliced)
- 1 banana (peeled)
- 1 cup unsweetened coconut milk or almond milk
- 1 tablespoon maple syrup (or other sweetener)
- 1 tablespoon virgin coconut oil
- ½ tablespoon unsweetened coconut flakes for the topping
- 1 teaspoon vanilla extract
- 1 teaspoon vanilla extract

Method:

1. Blend all the ingredients in your blender and sprinkle coconut flakes on the top of each serving

Pineapple and Strawberry Smoothie

A great smoothie though adjust the liquid levels to get the consistency you prefer.

Ingredients:

- 8oz frozen chopped pineapple
- 6oz frozen strawberries
- ¾ to 1 cup coconut milk
- 2 teaspoons coconut oil

Method:

1. Blend in your food process until smooth then serve garnished with a wedge of fresh pineapple

ENDNOTE

Coconut oil is a fantastic substance that has a huge amount of health benefits to you. Whilst it should never take the place of qualified medical advice, it can certainly compliment treatment and act as a preventative medicine. It is far better to take care of your body before it gets damaged or diseased.

With coconut oil being so full of vitamins, minerals and other beneficial substances it is something that more people should be using in their diets. With its ability to fight infection, reduce the signs of aging, aid digestion and help your body in so many ways it could help prevent many of the health problems people in the West face. Having been shown to lower cholesterol levels it can be a major contributor to the battle to prevent heart disease and high blood pressure.

The beauty applications of coconut oil are also significant because it is so nourishing for your skin and hair. It is applied to the skin and hair of many people who live where coconuts grow natively and you will find they all have luxurious, thick hair and very few signs of balding. For anyone who wants to take care of their hair or skin, coconut oil is perfect because it is one of the best products available and is not that expensive in its natural form. When you look at many commercially available beauty products, including shampoos, many of these contain coconut oil because it is so good for you.

In this book you have learnt all about the many applications of coconut oil and how to use it to help acne, for beauty purposes, on your hair plus how to cook with it and drink it.

Consuming coconut oil is a great way to gain many of the internal benefits of coconut oil though for beauty applications it is obviously best applied to the area. However, consuming coconut oil will still provide some benefit to your skin and hair!

Now you need to order yourself some coconut oil or go out and buy some and start using it in your everyday life. Use it in cooking instead of other oils, or use half olive oil (which has loads of health benefits) and half coconut oil. Try some of the recipes in this book and use some of the beauty applications. Whether you are male or female, coconut oil can help you look and feel fantastic!

With the shocking increase in preventable health issues in Western countries, using coconut oil can provide some much needed assistance in improving the health of the population. Whilst coconut oil is still relatively unheard of and used by relatively few people, it is gaining in popularity as people wake up to the health benefits of this oil and realize just how much it can benefit them.

Now enjoy using coconut oil and notice the difference to yourself when you use it. It is such a beneficial oil that everyone should be using it but now you know about it you can use it to improve your health, to look fantastic and to feel amazing!

OTHER BOOKS BY JENNY

Please check out my other health, cooking and beauty books on Amazon, available on Kindle and paperback. Get these books for free on Kindle Unlimited as part of your Amazon Prime membership.

Beauty

Luxurious Bath Bombs - 40 Bath Bomb Recipes: Simply DIY Recipes for Relaxation or Profit

Learn how to make your own luxurious bath bombs at home with these fantastic recipes for over 40 different, decadent bath bombs that turns bath time into a luxury, relaxing time. Discover the many different oils and ingredients you can use and how these can benefit your health, relax your muscles, help your skin and more. Click here now to find out how you can easily and cheaply be making your own amazing bath bombs at home.

Cooking

50 Meatball Recipes to Die For

Over 50 different meatball recipes that are mouth-wateringly delicious! Whether you like turkey, beef, pork or lamb meatballs you will find recipe after recipe here to impress your friends, win a cook-off or just enjoy a good meal. With sauce recipes too there is something here for everyone and you'll find this book packed full of recipes you can't wait to try! Click here now to preview this book.

99 Delicious Smoothie Recipes for A Healthier, Thinner You

Smoothies are a wonderful way to benefit from the vitamins, minerals and health boost from fruits and vegetables plus they are fantastic for anyone who is slimming. With 99 delicious recipes in this book you will be spoilt for choice and can find some great recipes you will love and enjoy! Click here now for a preview of the book

Cooking With Coffee - 40 Delicious Coffee Recipes For The Coffee Lover

Coffee is one of the most under-used and under-stated ingredients in cookery yet it makes for delicious desserts and mouth-watering main courses, locking in the flavor and giving a dish a rich, full taste. Find out why coffee is so good for you and how you can use it to make the tastiest meals ever with over 40 main courses, desserts and drinks that will blow your taste buds! Click here now to preview this book.

The Mediterranean Diet Cookbook - 100 Delicious Yet Healthy Mediterranean Diet Recipes

Proven to be probably the healthiest diet on the planet, the Mediterranean diet is one that promotes good health, long life and vitality! Discover the secrets of the Mediterranean people and how the food they eat benefits their health. Learn why the Western diet is so unhealthy and find out how you can enjoy these delicious and healthy recipes which will improve your health and help you to lose weight.

ABOUT THE AUTHOR

Jenny is passionate about heathy living and her realization of the importance of coconut oil for good health prompted her to write this book. She is keen for people to understand that the vegetable oils they use in their cooking are harmful to their health and that coconut oil has so many benefits for us all.